AT LAST . . . AN HONEST GUIDE TO GOOD EATING AND GOOD HEALTH!

"NUTRITION SCOREBOARD stands a good chance of being the most easily understood of all nutritional guidelines. . . ."   *Washington Star-News*

"Sometimes you want to know in a hurry just what food is really greatest in riboflavin . . . Or where the most niacin is . . . Most often, you crave word on how to have superb nutrition without a single excess calorie of any of those wrong fats. Where the facts are is . . . NUTRITION SCOREBOARD. . . ."   *Vogue*

Michael F. Jacobson, Ph.D., is co-director of the Center for Science in the Public Interest, a non-profit consumer advocacy organization. Jacobson, a microbiologist, is a former Nader worker and research associate of the Salk Institute. He is the author of EATER'S DIGEST, a fact book about food additives. He lives and works in Washington, D.C.

NUTRITION SCOREBOARD

YOUR GUIDE TO BETTER EATING

MICHAEL F. JACOBSON, PH.D.
Center for Science in
the Public Interest

AVON
PUBLISHERS OF BARD, CAMELOT, DISCUS, EQUINOX AND FLARE BOOKS

This is a revised and enlarged edition of NUTRITION SCOREBOARD

AVON BOOKS
A division of
The Hearst Corporation
959 Eighth Avenue
New York, New York 10019

ISBN: 0-380-00534-4

First Avon Printing, November, 1975

Printed in the U.S.A.

Some All-Star Foods

Liver, beef	2 oz.	**172**
Broccoli	3⅛ oz.	**116**
Cantaloupe	¼ melon	99
Cod, broiled	3 oz.	40
Milk, whole	8 oz.	39
Tomato juice	4 oz.	37
Rye bread	2 slices	29
Peanuts	¼ cup	25

Some Junkyard Foods

Soda pop	12 oz.	—92
Morton coconut cream pie	¼ pie	—62
Kool-Aid	8 oz.	—55
Jell-O	½ cup	—45
Del Monte vanilla pudding	1	—43
Candy bar, average	1 bar	—34
Hot dog	1	6

Avoid fat, sugar, white flour

Acknowledgements

It is a pleasure to thank publicly some of the many people who helped me prepare Nutrition Scoreboard.

James Silverman was an M.I.T. nutrition student when he worked with me at the Center for Science in the Public Interest (CSPI) as an intern. Jim helped me refine the food rating formula, and then calculated the scores of over two hundred foods, practically memorizing food composition tables in the process.

Alan Ackerman, Albert Fritsch, Mary Goodwin, Joan Gussow, Ogden Johnson, Sandra Kageyama, Stephen Kreitzman, James Sullivan, and my father, Larry Jacobson, read various drafts of this book and offered valuable criticisms and suggestions. Patti Hausman, my colleague at CSPI, did most of the research for the section on infant feeding.

Phyllis Machta deserves special thanks. She has spent many enjoyable hours carefully researching the medical literature, and has brought me a steady flow of interesting and important scientific articles. She, more than anyone, spurred my interest in the relationship between diet and disease.

I am delighted that the publication of the Avon edition of Nutrition Scoreboard *gives me an opportunity to thank some of the people who helped with the first edition, which was published in July, 1973, by CSPI. Robert White, my assistant at the time, did yeoman service in typing and otherwise preparing that edition* for publication. He also did some of the legal and other research that I refer to in this book as being done by CSPI. After the book came out, Phyllis Machta was a godsend in overseeing distribution of mail orders, and David Marcuse, of RPM Distributor, got Nutrition Scoreboard into bookstores. Many readers of the first edition sent me valuable ideas and suggestions, and I have incorporated many of these into this edition.

Sherry Donovan, Kathy Kahn, and Sam Abbott were the artists who designed the cover and provided illustrations for the first edition of Nutrition Scoreboard. Some of those illustrations are used in this edition.

To all these persons, and others not named, I give a hearty thanks!

MICHAEL F. JACOBSON
WASHINGTON, D.C.
JUNE, 1975

Contents

I. The American Way of Eating

PEOPLE WHO EAT brown rice and whole wheat bread are called food faddists, while children who gobble Fruity Pebbles and Sir Grapefellow are considered normal, red-blooded Americans. At a time when nutritionists and dentists are decrying diets high in sugar and refined flour, Betty Crocker and Sara Lee rely heavily on these ingredients and continue to be two of America's favorite cooks. When consumer advocates—their teeth glistening with silver fillings—recently criticized sugar-coated cereals, a hurt Kellogg Company, whose sales total only about one billion dollars a year, issued a self-pitying press release (August 1, 1974) complaining that "it is outrageous that fear-mongering consumerists continue to slander the Kellogg Company, and to frighten America's parents with impunity. The time has come for us to start fighting for our rights." Alice would feel quite at home in the wonderland of food company talk, manufactured foods, and food advertising.

Food is a fascinating subject. By examining our food supply from different perspectives, we can learn about economics, human behavior, politics, nutrition, farming, ecology, and toxicology. A comprehensive treatise on food would be monumental and would certainly tax to the breaking point the patience and intelligence of any mortal writer. For this volume, then, let us be satisfied with an overview of one of the most interesting aspects of food: nutrition and its relationship to health.

Nutrition is important, there's no doubt about it. Poorly nourished children will not grow as fast as their friends. Schoolwork is extra painful for the child whose stomach is growling all day. Children and adults both are afflicted by obesity. A malnourished woman may give birth to an underweight, sickly baby. An inadequate diet reduces one's resistance to disease, increases tooth decay, and can cause that tired, droopy feeling. George Briggs, Professor of Nutrition at the University of California at Berkeley, and Helen Ullrich, editor of the *Journal of Nutrition Education*, have estimated that "The annual costs to our country from hunger and ... personal mismanagement of food to the detriment of one's health is approximately 30 billion dollars."[1] As Dr. Wilbur Atwater, one of the world's first nutrition scientists, wrote back in 1894, "To make the most out of a man, to bring him up to the desirable level of productive capacity, to enable him to live as a man ought live, he must be well fed."[2]

The nutritional status of Americans has been studied often in recent years, and there is no longer any question that problems exist. Virtually all the surveys pointed to one or more nutritional problems in the segment of the population that was examined. In the most extensive of the studies, conducted in 1968-1970, the Department of Health, Education and Welfare surveyed thousands of people, particularly poor people, in ten states. The study is referred to as the Ten-State Nutrition Survey. The Survey indicated that "a significant proportion of the population surveyed was malnourished or was at high risk of developing nutritional problems." Blacks and Spanish-speaking Americans had more nutritional problems than whites, and poor people had more problems than the better off.

The U. S. Department of Agriculture also surveys Americans' eating habits periodically. The survey conducted in 1965 revealed that, despite an overall increase in personal income and standard of living, more people had poor diets in 1965 than in 1955. The fraction of American families with "poor" diets* rose from 15 percent to 21 percent. Poor nutrition existed both among the poor and the rich.

Although poor nutrition is traditionally thought of in terms of vitamin, mineral, and protein defi-

*A "poor" diet is one containing less than two-thirds of the Recommended Dietary Allowances—RDA—for one or more nutrients. The Food and Nutrition Board of the National Academy of Sciences, which sets the RDAs, says that the RDAs: ". . . will maintain good nutrition in practically all healthy persons in the United States. . . . The allowances are designed to afford a margin sufficiently above average physiological requirements to cover variations among practically all individuals in the general population . . . but they are not necessarily adequate to meet the additional requirements of persons depleted by disease, traumatic stresses, or prior dietary inadequacies."

Because the RDAs include a margin of safety, small deficiencies will usually not result in malnutrition and health problems.

ciencies, millions of Americans suffer another kind of malnutrition: too rich a diet—too many calories—which leads to obesity. Dr. Ogden Johnson, former Director of Nutrition of the Food and Drug Administration (FDA), has estimated that approximately forty million Americans are overweight. Statistical tables of the Metropolitan Life Insurance Company indicate that more than half the people in certain age groups are overweight.[3] One study showed that by age six obesity was nine times as prevalent among poor girls as among higher-income girls.[4]

People who are overweight have a greater than average likelihood of having a heart attack, developing high blood pressure, or suffering from diabetes. In addition, obese people often have tremendous social and psychological problems that can seriously hamper their chances for entering college, getting the desired job, and leading a happy, successful life. The tendency to eat too much is obviously encouraged by the relatively sedentary life style that urbanization and automation have made possible, and by the aggressive marketing of foods that are high in calories and low in nutrients, such as soda pop, candy, beer, and snack foods.

"Thirty percent of the products in grocery stores today could be thrown out and nobody would be the worse." Prof. D. Mark Hegsted, Dept. of Nutrition, Harvard School of Public Health, October 15, 1974.

In the United States we can define three broad classes of malnutrition. One kind is seen among the poor and exists largely because these people simply do not have enough money to buy adequate amounts and a good variety of food. Welfare recipients receive astonishingly little money for food. Montgomery County, Maryland is the nation's richest county, with an average family income of $23,000 a year. According to the County's nutritionist, Ms. Mary Goodwin, welfare recipients receive about 45 cents per person per meal, and only one-third that much if they do not get food stamps. Persons living in poverty may exhibit calorie, vitamin, mineral, and sometimes even protein deficiencies. As Margaret Mead has said, "The most important problems as I see it are to have both a nutritional program and enough food. I think it is important to realize that people don't eat nutrition. They eat food."[5]

Able-bodied men and women should have decent, and decent-paying, jobs; mothers, children, the infirm, and the aged should receive more money. Persons who are unemployed or receiving low incomes should ask their Mayor's office how to obtain food stamps. Millions of eligible persons are not taking advantage of this form of government assistance.

Some segments of the population have peculiar diets that lack certain, specific nutrients, and this is the second kind of malnutrition. Dedicated vegetarians may lack vitamin B-12 unless they take vitamin pills or eat dairy products. Women frequently do not eat enough iron-containing foods. Among some ethnic groups and in some regions of the country, diets may be deficient in vitamin A or

5

certain other nutrients. Correcting deficiencies of specific nutrients can sometimes be solved by a well-designed program of nutrition education.

The third kind of malnutrition is seen among all segments of the population, where diets contain too much of the wrong foods: sugar, starch, alcohol, and fat. These foods contribute little more than calories. Many of these malnourished people are overweight and destined to die of heart disease and stroke. These people—and this includes about one-half of all adults—might be awakened by an intensive and continuous education campaign geared to increase their awareness and understanding of foods and nutrition.

This third form of malnutrition is by far our greatest nutritional problem. Americans are suffereing incalculable pain, paying enormous medical costs, or dying prematurely because of illnesses such as diabetes, heart disease, and bowel cancer. These illnesses are occurring on an epidemic scale in Western nations and are caused, at least in part, by diet and other controllable factors. Most people assume that these serious illnesses are a natural and inescapable part of life, yet they are virtually unknown in some cultures. In short, these may be considered *unnecessary diseases*. (Particular diseases will be discussed in more detail later in this book.)

The unnecessary diseases develop slowly and quietly—not like measles or the chicken pox—and reflect the gradual disintegration of bodily organs and processes. They may begin in childhood, but not be manifest until old age. It is much harder for most people to be concerned about an unseen enemy that will not make its presence felt for twenty or thirty years than about an acute infectious disease—yet the two may be equally deadly. Understanding the long-term ill effects of our normal diet is the first step toward reducing the prevalence—and terrible personal and social costs—of the unnecessary diseases. The medical profession, too, could play a major role in stopping the epidemic, but it will have to shift its focus from *curing* diseases to *preventing* them.

If health considerations are not impressive enough to cause most people to change their diets, soaring food prices may be. Fortunately, the diet that is best for our health is also relatively inexpensive. Meat is the most expensive item in most of our food budgets—and, of course, it is also high in fat and cholesterol. Coca Cola is about the same price as milk—and has no real nutritional value, just lots of sugar. Milk or fruit juices are much better buys. Beans, lentils, and brown rice have doubled or tripled in price in the past two years, but they are still economical compared with the meat or cheese for which they can substitute in the diet.

When calculating the true cost of food, we should really include the long-term health consequences of a bad diet. Thus, whatever one spends at the dentist should be considered part of the food bill. A good part of the many billions of dollars we spend every year in treating diabetes, diverticulosis, constipation, and heart disease more properly belongs in the food budget than the health budget. If these costs could be calculated, they could be incorporated into the food price by taxing the

7

manufacturer and using the proceeds to help pay for health care. At the same time, the higher cost of less nutritious foods would discourage people from buying them.

In June, 1974, the Senate Select Committee on Nutrition and Human Needs sponsored a three-day National Nutrition Policy Study that brought together many of the nation's leading nutritionists, agricultural economists, public interest advocates, and food industry executives. The Panel on Nutrition and Health focused its attention on heart disease, obesity, diabetes, and similar health problems. The Panel said that, "a few simple changes in the American diet and habits of life could greatly reduce the number of people who acquire these diseases and may die from them." In its report, the Panel strongly recommended that Americans switch to a diet low in calories, saturated fat, sugar, cholesterol, and salt:

The "alternative diet" is designed to prevent disease and, at the same time, is nutritionally adequate. Because it is largely but not completely derived from legumes [pod vegetables: beans, peas, peanuts, etc.], grains, vegetable and fruit products, it is less expensive to produce in terms of resources than the present American diet based much more on food products derived from animals. It has this additional feature of ecological soundness at a time of world food shortages.

It is ironic that the richest people in the history of the world should have such widespread nutritional deficiencies and degenerative illnesses, while certain far more primitive populations have well-balanced diets and enjoy excellent health. A recent

article in *Science* magazine described the !Kung*
people, who have lived as hunters and gatherers in
the Kalahari Desert of South Africa for at least
11,000 years. Their diet:

consists of nuts, vegetables, and meat and lacks milk
and grains. All the investigators agree that the diet is
nutritionally well balanced and provides an adequate
number of calories. They found very few people with
iron deficiency anemia, even when they included pregnant and lactating women in their sample. . . . In
addition to being well nourished, the nomadic !Kung
are free from many common diseases.[6]

The researchers "have found little degenerative
disease among elderly !Kung, although it is com-
monplace for these people to live for at least 60
years and some live for as long as 80 years."[6]

Most of us have access to a much wider variety
of foods than the !Kung, but we have been uncon-
cerned about the nutritional value of what we
swallow. We consume a diet rich in meat, sugar,
and refined flour. This kind of diet is a novel experience for the human metabolism, which during
tens of thousands of years of evolution became ac-
customed to a diet more like the !Kung's. But there
have been holdouts, individuals and groups who
practice dietary conservatism and refuse to buy the
standard American fare so widely advertised on
television and readily available in supermarkets,
restaurants, and vending machines. Adherents to the
Seventh-Day Adventist faith provide an example
and can serve as America's control group. They eat
little meat, and thus have a relatively low-fat diet.

*The "!" represents a clicking sound.

Their diet is high in grains, fruits, and vegetables, and therefore relatively high in dietary fiber (sometimes called "roughage" or "bulk"). Strict adherents are vegetarians, non-smokers, and non-drinkers. Seventh-Day Adventists are remarkably healthy. According to one study, their death rate is 35 percent lower (in terms of deaths per 100,000 persons per year) than the rest of the population. The incidence of cirrhosis of the liver is 80 percent less than the rest of the population. They suffer 30 percent fewer deaths due to heart disease, and 25 percent fewer deaths due to cancer. The risk of death due to mouth and lung cancer is half as great among Seventh-Day Adventists as the rest of the population.[7] The remarkable contrast between Seventh-Day Adventists and the general population would have been even greater if only strict adherents to the Seventh-Day Adventist way of life were included in the study.

The sound nutritional advice offered by the Panel on Nutrition and Health got a line or two in the newspapers back in June, 1974, but it probably did not cause many people to change their eating habits. Advice about nutrition, to be effective, must be backed by a well-financed and executed educational campaign. But nutrition education in the United States is dead. Actually, it's worse than dead, because most of the information that we get about foods and nutrition comes from the food industry, and it is no secret that much of that industry—like any other industry—is more concerned with the size of its profits than about the public's intake of nutrients.

For the past twenty-five years the public has

10

learned most of what it knows about food from advertising. Tony the Tiger has been hammering into our children's heads, with machine-gun frequency and ferocity, that Kellogg's Sugar Frosted Flakes are Grrrrrrrrreat. (According to *Advertising Age*, Kellogg spent more than $4.5 million advertising Frosted Flakes in 1973.[8]) The food industry spends over $4 billion a year on advertising. This advertising has been our teacher and has had a great impact on our eating habits.

But don't schools teach nutrition? Remember your home economics class in junior high? Did you ever wonder where our teachers got their information and colorful wall posters about foods? There is a paperback book by Thomas J. Pepe entitled *Free and Inexpensive Educational Aids* (Dover Publications) which is intended primarily for teachers. In the section on nutrition and diet, 157 booklets, charts, movies, and leaflets are offered. The food industry sponsors 154 of these, a life insurance company one, and the U.S. Department of Agriculture (USDA) two. From the Pickle Packers International, Inc., to the National Macaroni Institute, the information comes pouring forth, each industry shouting the glorious virtues of its products. Some of the information is accurate and responsible, some is subtly deceptive, and some is downright laughable. Many teachers, unfortunately, rely extensively on this, the most easily available information, to supplement standard texts.

The National Confectioners Association, which represents the makers of $3 billion worth of candy a year (1.5 billion pounds of sugar are used in this candy), will supply any teacher with plenty of pro-candy propaganda. One of the Association's booklets, "The Story of Candy," extols candy's "ability to furnish energy, fight fatigue and fever, curb oversized appetites, and all the rest" (which includes relieving growing pains and preventing diarrhea and convulsions), and also tells us that candy can "work to depress the appetite and act as an aid to the weight-watcher." (In 1972 the Federal Trade Commission forced the sugar industry to correct deceptive advertisements by running new ads saying "Research hasn't established that consuming sugar before meals will contribute to weight reduction or even keep you from gaining weight.") The American Medical Association, American Dental Association and the National Institute of Dental Research all agree that sugar in general, and candy in particular, contribute to tooth decay—especially when it is consumed between meals, as the candy industry recommends for weight-watchers.

Even the soft drink industry, which pushes its liquid junk with unflagging fervor, manages to find health benefits in its product. After bragging about the energy-providing (their euphemism for calories) sugar, the National Soft Drink Association reminds us, in a booklet entitled "The Story of Soft Drinks," that soda pop is a great source of water! The soft drink is also said to help settle upset stomachs, and "to provide a psychological lift and ... ease some of the day's tensions." (Actually, colas and Dr. Pepper contain caffeine and may *increase* the day's tensions.) Soft drinks supply calories, but no vitamins, minerals, or protein. They displace nutritious foods from our diet. In 1973 the

Coca Cola Company's $76 million advertising budget was about 15 percent larger than the entire budget of the FDA's Bureau of Foods. (See Appendix I for a listing of the advertising budgets of major food producers.)

The Pickle Packers International, Inc., offers a lively 16-page booklet, "New Facts about an Old Friend," extolling the nutritional value of the pickle. "Nutritive elements which pickles contain in generous measure ... vitamin A? Yes, indeed ... [pickles] also provide some B-1 and B-2 and a *considerable amount of the important vitamin C.*" In fact, the pickle is one of the least nutritious vegetables. A 2⅛ ounce pickle contains only 1.5 percent of the RDA (Recommended Daily Allowance) of vitamin A, just a trace of vitamin B-1, 1 percent of the RDA of vitamin B-2, and 7 percent of the RDA of vitamin C. The pickle may taste good, but telling school children that it is highly nutritious is downright dishonest.

A major source of nutrition materials for teachers is the National Dairy Council. This industry group has prepared posters, movies, booklets, and many other items. In fact, so earnest is the Dairy Council that it has come to consider nutrition education its turf, according to some nutritionists. In California, the Dairy Council stood on the sidelines while apparently more concerned nutritionists fought for—but did not get—a state-supported nutrition education program. Much of the Dairy Council's educational arsenal is accurate and well-prepared. However, problems associated with the over-consumption of fat and cholesterol (which are present in milk, cream, and ice cream) are rarely

13

discussed. Also, as one would expect from an industry group, the materials never go beyond the strictest boundaries, and never touch on the politics of nutrition: TV advertising aimed at selling junk foods to children, deficiencies in Federal regulatory agencies, and hunger and malnutrition in America. This omission would be excusable were it not that the Dairy Council virtually monopolizes the field of nutrition education and many teachers know of no other source of information about the underlying causes of bad nutrition.

In the classroom, children *hear* what society says about nutrition; in the school cafeteria, children *eat* foods that show what society really thinks about nutrition. The cafeteria should be a showplace of good nutrition and a living example of nutrition education. But, alas, the opportunity has been lost, despite the increasingly heavy involvement—and potential for influence—of the Federal Government in school feeding programs. The most egregious product in school food lines is the USDA-approved vitamin-fortified cake, which may contain as much as 30 percent sugar. "Astrofood" is the name of ITT-Continental Baking's contribution to the school breakfast program. A complete breakfast consists of a cake and a glass of milk. Is it any wonder that after a government-approved, school-sanctioned breakfast like this students consider cakes and snacks of all kinds to be a reasonable way to get nourishment? Fortunately, few schools are using vitamin-fortified cakes. At lunch children are tempted with potato chips, cookies, doughnuts, fruit drinks (instead of juices), and other goodies. Between classes, students in many schools can buy soda pop and candy from vending machines in the corridors. The U.S. Congress recently passed legislation to permit vending machines right in school cafeterias. While the machines could offer milk, nuts, fruit, and other nutritious products, it is almost inevitable that most will dispense candy, gum, soda pop, and cookies. In 1972 Lawrence Hogan, who was then Congressman from Maryland, said that it would be "unfortunate" if soft drinks were banned from these machines.[9] Nutrition educators have a long way to go.

Governmental agencies at the state, city, and federal levels could and should be providing the public with a steady flow of interesting and hard-hitting nutrition information, but they barely give this topic lip service. The Federal effort, conducted primarily by the Department of Agriculture, is hampered by a lack of funds and lack of desire and by political pressures. General Mills spent over $6 million in 1973 on Cheerios advertising—this figure dwarfs the Federal expenditure for nutrition education, which is no more than $2 million (although this depends on just how "nutrition education" is defined). The companies that have millions of dollars to spend on product advertising have similar resources for influencing legislators. Any government-sponsored nutrition message that takes

"We've let the food manufacturers into our kitchens. Now they should let us into their board rooms." Esther Peterson, President, National Consumers League.

even the meekest of pokes at a big industry is likely to have a very short life. Despite the general recognition that sugar causes tooth decay, the sugar industry and food manufacturers which produce sugared products will simply not permit an anti-sugar campaign. Research, yes; public education, no. Thus, the National Institute of Dental Research has a $43 million budget, but only $40,000 (0.1 percent) is earmarked for public education. That saturated fat and cholesterol contribute to heart disease suggests the importance of conducting a campaign urging people to eat less meat and eggs (two major sources of fat and cholesterol). After all, shouldn't our Department of Health, Education and Welfare, as well as our Department of Agriculture's nutrition section, inform us of measures we could take to improve our health? But the farming and ranching interests are powerful. HEW has said nothing, USDA booklets tell us how to cook eggs, and in June, 1974, Secretary of Agriculture Earl Butz told us to stock up on meat. Our Government will provide us with health information, but only if it does not conflict with the interests of a major industry. Unfortunately, good advice about nutrition conflicts with the interests of many big industries, each of which has more lobbying power than all the public-interest groups combined.

The excellent health status of the Seventh-Day Adventists indicates the value of good nutrition and suggests that a careful study to determine the effectiveness of a massive nutrition education program would be a worthwhile investment. Because heart disease, tooth decay, diabetes, bowel cancer, and several other health problems appear to be caused, at least in part, by diet, an effective nutrition education campaign should cause measurable reductions in the incidences of these illnesses. The campaign should focus on encouraging the public to eat a low-fat, low-sugar, low-salt, low-cholesterol, high-fiber diet. The diet would be relatively low in foods of animal origin and high in foods of vegetable origin. The diet in no way resembles a faddist diet, and any health risks associated with it would be miniscule.

Small to medium sized towns should be invited to vie for the honor of being testing grounds for "health promoting diets" (HPD). In the fortunate towns chosen for this unique effort, resources would be mobilized to encourage the public to eat the healthful diet. Necessary funding and overall direction would come from the Department of Health, Education and Welfare. Radio and TV stations would broadcast spot announcements and programs pertaining to nutrition and health. Supermarket displays and ads would encourage shoppers to buy nutritious foods. School teachers and children would learn about the benefits of the HPD. The towns' health departments would use movies, literature, and the mass media to advocate good eating habits. The vending-machine operators and restaurant owners would encourage their patrons, by means of wider choices and more education, to eat foods characteristic of the HPD. Fruits, vegetables, whole wheat bread, and low-fat milk would be made as readily available in the town as soft

17

drinks and candy are today. Advertising of non-nutritious foods on television would be sharply curtailed. Obviously, a vigorous campaign to encourage good eating habits would run into stiff commercial opposition, but hopefully there are a few towns whose merchants would make some sacrifices to allow their town to achieve a place of distinction in the annals of public health.

A concerted effort to improve diet could have a major impact within two or three years, despite the fact that many diseases take years or decades to develop. For instance, during World War II the incidence of diabetes in Britain declined sharply, probably due to changes in diet. Also, the probability of lung cancer drops quickly when a smoker kicks the habit.

During the campaign to promote dietary changes, physicians, statisticians, and epidemiologists would monitor the disease and mortality rates and compare them to the rates prior to the study period. Changes in food consumption could be measured by supermarket sales records and diet-recall surveys.

A study of this magnitude would obviously re-

"We have simply not given a fraction of the time, talent and resources to the prevention of malnutrition that we have to the experimental studies for the acquisition of nutritional knowledge." Dr. Nevin Scrimshaw, Chairman, M.I.T. Dept. of Nutrition and Food Science, 1972.

quire a great pooling of professional resources, but the unique potential for improving the public's health would be well worth the expense. If disease rates are, indeed, cut because of the intervention, the method could be used to encourage the HPD nationwide. The scores or hundreds of lives saved in the several small towns could lead to the saving of tens of thousands of lives in the nation at large. The cost of this study would be an amount far less than the amount any big food company spends on advertising.

Although the Federal government has been reticent about providing nutrition information, few others have been shy and the public has the problem of knowing just who to believe. Nutrition is an extraordinarily broad subject and no one expert can possibly have a deep knowledge of more than a few areas. Because food companies and the nutritionists who work for them obviously have vested interests, one often turns to the academic community for straight answers. But caution must be exercised here, too, because professors are not always as unbiased as one would assume. One problem is that scientists often exaggerate the significance of their own research or area of specialization. A more obvious and serious problem is that companies frequently hire nutrition professors as consultants, or dispense research grants, or serve as potential employers of a professor's students. Many academic food experts develop close ties with food, drug, and chemical companies and are financially rewarded. There is nothing illegal about this practice, but professors who also work for food companies should not expect the public to consider them to be completely unbiased sources of information. Further, it is not always possible for the public to discover from which outside sources a professor has received income or favors.

The most well-known friend of industry in the academic nutrition world is Dr. Frederick Stare. Stare, who has conducted important diet-heart studies, is chairman of the Department of Nutrition at the Harvard School of Public Health. At a time when hundreds of health professionals and professional organizations have been attacking the over-consumption of table sugar and sugar-coated cereals, Stare has been vigorously defending these foods. At the highly publicized 1970 Congressional hearings on breakfast cereals, Stare maintained that "sugar added to cereals does not cause any deterioration of the nutritional qualities of the cereal. . . ."[10] More recently, he was quoted in an interview as saying that "most people could healthily double their sugar intake daily."[11] Is it just a coincidence that he has received retainers from Kellogg, Nabisco, and the Cereal Institute (the breakfast cereal companies' trade association)?[12] He has also testified at FDA hearings on behalf of the Sugar Association, Carnation Milk, Pharmaceutical Manufacturers Association, and the Cereal Institute. In late 1974, Stare refused to disclose to the author the organizations for which he was then consulting.

The Harvard School of Public Health building, which houses Stare's department, bears a plaque thanking General Foods Corporation for its generosity in making possible the nutrition research laboratories. Some of the other organizations that have helped support the department, but that did not rate plaques, include Beech-Nut, Kellogg, Sugar Association, Procter & Gamble, and Nabisco. Generous gifts are often repaid in one way or another.

The manufacturers of infant formula and baby food have given grants to many researchers in the field of pediatric nutrition. This generosity has promoted close ties between the scientists and the companies and has successfully nipped most potential criticism in the bud.

A cozy relationship between a professor and a food corporation does not necessarily mean that the professor has prostituted himself or herself, but all too often that appears to be the case. Industrial ties neutralize critics. Friends of companies often distort evidence or offer carefully selected facts. They tend to ask the public to prove that a food or chemical is hazardous rather than demand that the manufacturer demonstrate that it is safe. These professors always seem to find some way of excusing even the most egregious products (like

Note to nutritionists: "In my opinion, you have a choice. Either you are committed to better nutrition for the American people . . . or you can retreat to the safety of the laboratory or clinic or hide among the bureaucracy of the established, special interest groups representing the largely monetary motivated interests of industry, medicine, and agriculture." Dr. Hermann Bleibtreu, Professor of Anthropology, University of Arizona, 1972.

baby food desserts and candy-like cereals) or corporate policies (like high-pressure advertising aimed at children). The big food companies that offer grants and consulting fees are the major producers and advertisers of junk foods, and they seem to have the most friends in the academic community. Manufacturers of "health foods" and "natural foods," on the other hand, are fair game. They are outside of the fraternity and their very existence is an implied criticism of the major companies. (This is not to say that the health food and vitamin companies are without fault; their advertising is sometimes extremely deceptive.) While we do not argue that companies should not receive the advice of academic experts, we do question the ethics of the professors who accept payment (in dollars or in favors) for their advice. This is especially true of professors in state-supported institutions, who are paid a salary by the taxpayers to work full-time. At the very least, professors who receive corporate money should be required by law to make this information public. Reporters should always ask their academic sources for this information. Knowing who pays the piper will help us decide who is calling the tune.

Aggressive, creative, well-funded nutrition education campaigns may be exercises in futility unless they are accompanied by actions on other fronts. The giant food corporations, which are churning out bad food along with the good, must be more strictly controlled—by citizen pressure, competitive pressures, and government regulations. The ubiquitous vending machine, that mute metallic purveyor of junk, is undergoing a population explosion that should be checked. Advertising should be banned from television programs aimed at children, and more stringently controlled in other areas. The sugar content of certain foods

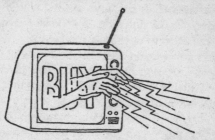

should be limited by law and disclosed on food labels. In short, this country needs a national nutrition policy. For far too long we have defaulted and allowed corporations to set nutrition policy in a way that increases private wealth at the expense of public health.

Availability is a powerful, but rarely acknowledged, influence on our eating habits. Unfortunately, as the United States becomes more advanced technologically, it is becoming more limited nutritionally. As we eat more of our meals outside of the home, it is getting harder and harder to obtain nutritious foods. Supermarkets, despite their vast size, often do not carry such basic commodities as brown rice and whole wheat flour. Rural grocery stores rarely seem to carry whole wheat bread. White bread is often doctored with caramel coloring to make it look like whole wheat bread. Green vegetables seem to be *persona non grata* in fast-food restaurants. The refreshment stand in the shadow of the Washington Monument—and just a few blocks from the White House, the Department of Agriculture, and the Food and Drug Administration—specializes in junk foods. Last time I dropped in they had only hot dogs, soda pop, non-carbonated soft drinks and candy. Understanding the principles of nutrition is little use if one does not have access to nutritious foods.

When government surveys show that millions of Americans are poorly nourished, food industry executives blame the consumer, saying that Americans do not shop wisely. This is exactly what industry has tried to do with regard to pollution: blame the individual for littering in order to distract attention from the wholesale manner in which corporations defile the earth, air, and water. The executives who decry nutritional ignorance are often the same ones who produce and promote junk foods. But the problem is not just the executives in the institutions, rather it is the very nature of the institutions themselves. As long as corporations continue to exist as they do today—acting according to self-interest instead of society's best interest—citizens will be forced to fend off ceaseless pressures to buy unwholesome food. Society's goal must be to maximize health, not profits.

The Food and Drug Administration (FDA) and the U.S. Department of Agriculture (USDA) are charged with regulating the food industry. But many of the top officials in these agencies are former food industry executives, and it would be naive to expect them to be strong critics or strict regulators of industry. Before he became Secretary of Agriculture, Earl Butz was a paid director of Ralston Purina. Dr. Virgil Wodicka, who recently resigned his position as FDA's Director of the Bureau of Foods, formerly worked for Hunt-Wesson; Libby, McNeill & Libby; and Ralston Purina. A survey taken by the Center for Science in the Public Interest in 1973, showed that twenty-two of fifty-two top posts in FDA were held by men and women who were formerly associated with regulated industry and other special-interest groups.[13] Not a single high-ranking FDA official has worked with a consumer group. If we ever hope to revitalize our food supply, this lopsided representation in government agencies must end.

Leaving FDA is another problem. The most lucrative positions for departing FDA officials are in the companies which FDA is supposed to regulate. In 1969, a Congressional committee discovered that thirty-seven of forty-nine recently resigned or retired employees went on to serve regulated industries in various capacities. In August, 1972, the Deputy Commissioner of FDA quit to become special

---

What Vending Machines Don't Vend: "Food contributes to physical, mental, and emotional health. Food nourishes our bodies. When we eat in a favorable setting, we get another kind of well-being: A sense of belonging and other psychological and social values accrue from the pleasures of mealtime and from having our food with friendly companions." U.S. Department of Agriculture, **1959 Yearbook.**

assistant to the Chairman of CPC, International, which makes Mazola margarine, Skippy peanut butter, and Hellman's mayonnaise, among other products. He took with him to his new employer useful contacts in FDA and full knowledge of all of FDA's future plans. In March, 1974, Dr. Ogden Johnson, FDA's Director of Nutrition, departed for greener pastures: Hershey Corporation, maker of candy and chocolate syrup. How is the public to trust its regulatory officials if they are fishing for jobs with the very companies they are paid to regulate? Some of these job transfers between government and industry are listed in Appendix II.

While we are primarily interested in the nutritional effects of foods, we should not forget that foods and meals have traditionally served important social and psychological roles in our lives. The life style of Americans has changed dramatically in the last thirty years and with it our eating habits. The pace of our lives has become increasingly frenetic. Most people don't even make time to treat themselves to a good breakfast, but settle for a cup of coffee, doughnut, and cigarette. More and more foods are of the instant variety, what with toaster-tarts and drink mixes for breakfast, vending-machine sandwiches and beverages for lunch, and frozen dinners for supper. The availability of these convenience foods has aided and abetted the disappearance of the family meal, as has the increasing proportion of women who work. The exodus of young families to suburbia has stranded many elderly people who must now shift for themselves or rely on government programs for food and companionship.

Although new food additives are now tested for adverse physiological effects, new foods are not being studied for adverse sociological and psychological effects. But they must be, because we are rapidly headed for a 1984-like Nutri-pill, which will contain all of our known nutritional requirements. The food industry is hellbent in this direction. Breakfast cereals fortified with 100 percent of our daily requirement of ten nutrients, Space Stick candy bars, and Instant Breakfasts offer a glimpse of the future, and the food technologists are working feverishly in their laboratories, developing "newer and better" concoctions. A vending machine dispensing Nutri-pills may be the dinner table of tomorrow. We must stop and ask ourselves if we really prefer missing out on the social opportunity that a family meal offers. Foods have served

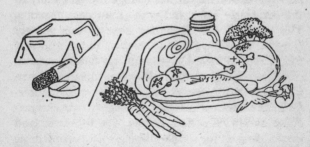

as a link between nature and man. The supermarket is already a far cry from a farm. Are we really ready to take the next step and dissociate nutrients completely from the animal or vegetable sources from which we have obtained them for hundreds of thousands of years? Is a rubber nipple and glass bottle an adequate substitute for the human breast

27

and a mother's warmth? Questions like these deserve careful study by sociologists, psychiatrists, and psychologists. While they study, however, the food industry will be churning out new foods and new "food concepts." Therefore, it is urgent that we consider the role of foods and eating in our lives—before every shopping trip and before every meal. Food is too important to be left to the food industry.

I hope this introduction has highlighted the enormously beneficial value of eating a good diet and the influences that are discouraging most of us from getting that diet. I have tried to emphasize the dietary changes most of us should concentrate on: eating more vegetable foods, less fat-laden meat, and fewer sugary, salty, greasy snack foods. The principles of a good diet are really quite simple. One does not have to read a hundred books or make the study of foods the whole focus of one's life to understand these principles. But considering how important good nutrition is for our health, and considering that we eat a thousand meals and perhaps another thousand snacks a year, is it unreasonable to devote perhaps a day or two of one's life to studying nutrition in order to understand clearly a few life-saving rules? Once we integrate these rules into our lives, we can stop worrying about the composition of our diet and spend our time on more interesting and challenging matters.

I receive many letters from people who say that *Nutrition Scoreboard* has helped them and their family or friends eat better. Often they want to know what they can do to help improve the nutritional quality of foods at the store and the eating habits of the public. My immediate and unqualified response is to urge them to fight the forces that are promoting bad nutrition. The best way to go about this is to join, start, or support a citizens action group. Define a problem that you are concerned about, and then go to work and try to solve it. Fight for better foods in your school cafeteria; get your local TV and radio stations to run pro-nutrition spots; press the Health Department to require that wherever foods are vended from machines, at least half the choices should be nourishing. If you're not a joiner, work alone for better food. Mrs. Jean Farmer of Bloomington, Indiana, is one such one-person army. She recently won a two-year battle to get junk foods banned from her county's school system. If you are too busy to work actively with a consumer group, support them financially. Most of them are perpetually broke and desperate for funds. The operating budgets of all consumer groups in the United States would not add up to the advertising budget of a single big food company. Cooperate with other activist groups, be enthusiastic, persevere; and above all: do it!

II. Rating the Nutritional Value of Food

THERE ARE TWO common ways of communicating information about the nutritive value of foods. One approach is to recite truthful generalities about foods, such as "we should eat a protein source at every meal," or "this or that food is rich in this or that vitamin." The Basic Four (protein foods, dairy products, grains, fruits and vegetables) approach to nutrition is in this vein—the good foods are given a pat on the back, while the bad foods are ignored. As government nutrition surveys (and sales figures for soda pop and snack foods) prove, this approach has not been successful in making good nutrition habits important to Americans.

The second popular approach is almost diametrically opposed to the first. Where the first offers generalities, the second chokes on details. Some government publications and some cookbooks have page after page of nutritional analyses of foods. The plethora of numbers is enough to scare off any but the most dedicated pursuers of information. Listed in the tables are the actual quantities of fat, protein, vitamins, and minerals contained in foods. With all the numbers, it requires a great effort to determine what constitutes a serving, whether that amount makes a significant contribution to the person's diet, and how one food compares to another. Expressing the data on a per-serving basis (rather than per-100 grams) and listing it as a percentage of the RDA helps some. But huge tables can be terribly confusing, and they are almost useless to most of us.

The Adelle Davis approach to nutrition is a complicated variation of this second approach. Her books detail the amount of each nutrient in each food, and discuss possible health benefits or hazards of the nutrients. This approach—making nutrition a study—has attracted hundreds of thousands of followers, perhaps as much as 2 percent of the population, and has sparked much of today's widespread concern about food quality. But the other 98 percent does not want to preoccupy itself with foods and health and could well benefit from a simpler approach to nutrition.

In 1961, Dr. Robert Harris, who was then a Professor (now Professor Emeritus) of Nutrition and Food Science at M.I.T., developed a new way of conveying information about the nutritional value of food. He and his colleagues analyzed the composition of forty-four different kinds of bread.[14] He than ranked each bread according to how much of each of fourteen different nutrients it contained, averaged the rankings of each bread, and gave each bread a "nutritional rating." He listed the breads in a table, the best (by his scoring system) being No. 1 and the worst being No. 44. By calculating a single number for each bread, he could rank breads in order, running from best to worst.

This system saves the reader all the trouble of comparing each bread for each nutrient, and offers at a glance the important information: which are the most nutritious breads, which are the least nutritious. His secret was to reduce the number of nutritional variables from fourteen (in the case of bread) to one.

The same approach was used in 1970 by Robert Choate (who has been prominent in the battle to restrict TV advertising aimed at children) to rate the nutritional value of breakfast cereals. He presented his easy-to-understand ratings at a Congressional hearing, and the next day they were front-page news in newspapers across the country. People could tell at a glance which were the best cereals (according to Choate's criteria) and which were the worst. Choate's system had several serious shortcomings, but the ease with which his simple ratings communicated nutrition information helped make the public aware of nutrition and caused cereal companies to add vitamins and minerals to many of the cereals that were near the bottom of this chart.[15]

One problem with Choate's system was that vitamin-fortified cereals had high ratings, and were therefore "good," even when they contained 40 percent sugar and were sprayed with artificial coloring and flavoring. This suggested that if simple ratings were to be meaningful, foods that got credit for the good things in them should also be penalized for ingredients that can be unhealthful. For example, Kaboom, a mixture of marshmallow bits and artificially colored, sugary oat clumps (made by General Mills), was tied for first place in Choate's chart. A product like Kaboom is nutritious—it is essentially a sugar-coated vitamin pill—but it is more a candy than a cereal and should not be sitting at the top of any nutrition chart.

Nutrition Scoreboard takes the same general approach that Mr. Choate used to rate cereals and that Professor Harris used to rate breads, but it has several refinements and we apply it to many kinds of foods. The formula that we have developed gives a food credit for some of its nutritious ingredients, and deducts credit for substances that Americans frequently eat too much of. The substances that get positive credit are:

- Protein
- Naturally occurring carbohydrate (including starch, fiber, glycogen [animal starch], and sugars)
- Vitamins A, B-1 (or B-6), B-2, B-3 (niacin), C
- Iron and calcium (or magnesium)
- Trace minerals
- Unsaturated fat

The substances that are frequently consumed in excess and for which we subtract points are:

- Sugar (and corn syrup) that is added to food
- Saturated fat
- High fat content

None of these ingredients are inherently bad, and for many people moderate amounts pose no threat. But for the average, urban, sedentary American, the amount of these substances currently consumed

34

increase the risk of developing a variety of illnesses.

As an example of how the formula works, here are breakdowns of the ratings of a 3-ounce hamburger and a Milky Way candy bar:

Hamburger		Milky Way Candy Bar	
Protein	20	Protein	3.1
Carbohydrate	0	Carbohydrate, natural added sugar, and corn syrup	2.8
			−47.5
Fat: quantity	−8.4	Fat: quantity	0
quality	−4.7	quality	−3.9
Vitamins: A	0.3	Vitamins: A	1.3
B-1	2.3	B-1	1
B-2	5.3	B-2	4
B-3	11.5	B-3	0
C	0	C	0.5
Minerals: iron	7.5	Minerals: iron	1
calcium	0.5	calcium	4.5
Total	34.3	Total	−33.2

Each factor in the formula used to rate the nutritional values of foods is discussed below. The rating for a food is obtained by adding the scores of all the factors. The coefficients in each factor were selected after carefully considering the health effects of the ingredients. The values for Recommended Daily Allowances (RDA)* are those chosen by the FDA for the purposes of nutrition labeling. (Recommended Daily Allowances set by FDA are slightly different from the Recommended Dietary

*Recommended Daily Allowances (U.S.) for persons over 4 years of age.

| Protein | 65 | grams[a] |
| Vitamin A | 5000 | units |

Allowances set by the National Academy of Sciences.) Calculations are done on a per-serving basis, rather than per-ounce, per-hundred grams, or per-calorie basis, because we are interested in how much nourishment there is in the portion of food that we actually eat. Information about the nutritional values and composition of the foods was obtained from companies, food packages, government publications, and by our own calculations.

Fiber
Linoleic Acid
Inositol
Choline
Potassium

Thiamin (vitamin B-1)	1.5	milligrams
Riboflavin (vitamin B-2)	1.7	milligrams
Niacin (vitamin B-3)	20	milligrams
Pyridoxine (vitamin B-6)	2	milligrams
Vitamin B-12	6	micrograms
Vitamin C	60	milligrams
Calcium	1	gram
Iron	18	milligrams
Magnesium	400	milligrams
Folic acid	0.4	milligrams
Pantothenic acid	10	milligrams
Biotin	0.3	milligrams
Vitamin D	400	units
Vitamin E	30	units
Phosphorus	1	gram
Iodine	150	micrograms
Zinc	15	milligrams
Copper	2	milligrams

ᵃIf the protein quality is equal to or better than that of casein (milk protein), the U.S. RDA is 45 grams.

Protein

$$\text{protein score} = 50 \times \frac{\text{grams of protein/serving} \times (\text{NPU}/100)^{\frac{1}{2}}}{43.1 \text{ grams}}$$

where NPU is a measure of protein quality

Protein, the stuff of which muscle, enzymes, hair, and cellular structures are made, is absolutely essential in a good diet. Protein deficiency is not a problem in the United States. If anything, our diets, being rich in meat and dairy products, contain too much protein.

Proteins are made up of amino acids linked end to end in long chains, much like cars in a long freight train. There are twenty different amino acids (analogous to twenty kinds of freight cars), and the number of each variety and the specific order in which they are linked is characteristic of each protein. The body can produce some, but not all, of the amino acids. The "essential amino acids"—those which the body cannot produce—must be obtained from food. Different proteins are of different value to the body, depending upon how much of the various amino acids they contain. The best quality protein occurs in egg, milk, and cheese; soy and meat proteins are also excellent. The protein of these foods is rich in the essential amino acids. Relatively poor quality protein occurs in some vegetables, like beans and peas. This protein contains relatively small amounts of one or more of the eight essential amino acids. The lowest quality, almost worthless, protein is gelatin. A person whose diet is high in poor quality protein must consume more protein than one whose diet is rich in eggs, dairy products, meat, and soy.

The number of points a food gets for protein is based on the percentage of the adult RDA of usable protein that the food supplies. The RDA for protein is 65 grams. This is slightly more than two ounces (one ounce contains 28.35 grams) of pure protein. However, because proteins contain different mixtures of amino acids, all proteins are not equally valuable. An average adult would need to consume only 43.1 grams of protein a day if that protein were of the highest quality. In other words, 43.1 grams of "perfect" quality protein is equivalent to 65 grams of average protein. The amount of "usable protein" in a food is the number of grams of total protein multiplied by a measure of protein quality. The measure of quality that we use is "net protein utilization" (NPU); we divide the NPU by 100 to obtain values betwen 0.0 and 1.0.

Proteins with different amino acid compositions complement one another if eaten at approximately the same time (within several hours). That is, an essential amino acid that is in short supply in one food may be supplied to the body by another food. This concept is explained clearly and at length in Frances Moore Lappé's exquisite book *Diet for a*

Small Planet, (Ballantine Books, 1971). Thus, a mixture of different foods in the diet usually results in an amino acid mixture that is more balanced than that of any of the component foods. To account for this apparent improvement in protein quality, the square root of NPU/100 rather than NPU/100 itself is used in our formula. *Diet for a Small Planet* lists the NPUs of many protein-containing foods. The points for protein that some foods receive are listed in Scoreboard 1.

SCOREBOARD 1

Protein Sources
(the average person needs 50 points per day)

Food	Serving Sizes	Protein Score*
Flounder, baked	3 oz.	28
Cod, broiled	3 oz.	27
Turkey, flesh	3 oz.	26
Chicken, breast	3 oz.	26
Tuna fish, packed in oil	3 oz.	25
Round steak, lean and fat	3 oz.	23
Pot roast	3 oz.	22
Hamburger, lean	3 oz.	22
Sirloin steak	3 oz.	18
Roast ham**	3 oz.	17
Cottage cheese	½ cup	16
Salmon, canned	3 oz.	16
Swiss cheese	2 oz.	15

Food	Serving Sizes	Protein Score*
American cheese	2 oz.	14
Liver, beef or chicken	2 oz.	14
Eggs	2 large	14
Beef stew, canned	1 cup	14
Pork sausage	2 links	12
Campbell Chunky Beef soup	1 cup	12
Shrimp, boiled	1½ oz.	11
Soybeans	½ cup	10
Milk	1 cup	9
Peanut butter	2 Tbsp.	7
Hot dog**	1	5
Macaroni	¾ cup	5
Special K	1 oz.	5

*Double these numbers to determine the percentage of RDA for protein that a food contributes to the diet.

**These foods contain sodium nitrite, an additive that should be avoided.

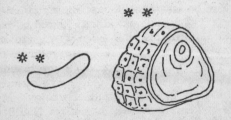

Carbohydrate

carbohydrate score = 50 ×

$$\frac{\text{grams of naturally occurring carbohydrate/serving}}{335 \text{ grams}}$$

+ 2 (grams of fiber/serving) − 2.5 (grams of added sugar/serving)

The carbohydrate factor includes three terms, one for each of three kinds of carbohydrate. The first term is the contribution that a food's naturally

> **"Where will the money come from to fund development of programs and materials [for nutrition education]? We suggest taxes be levied on those "empty calorie" foods such as soft drinks, candy, and snacks that contain little or no nutrient value, somewhat in the same manner as alcohol and tobacco products are taxed."**
> Dr. George Briggs, Professor of Nutrition, University of California, Berkeley; Ms. Helen Ullrich, Editor, Journal of Nutrition Education, 1972.

occurring carbohydrate makes to our nutritional needs.* This includes only the starch, sugar, or other carbohydrate that is naturally present in a food. Refined sugar or corn syrup that is added to food is not included.

Somehow starchy foods have gotten an ill-deserved reputation in recent years for being fattening. Bananas, potatoes, and whole wheat bread are all rich in starch, but the starch is accompanied by vitamins, minerals, and protein. The starch in natural foods is a good source of calories. Purified starch, however, offers nothing but calories when added to foods.

The second term is for dietary fiber (also called "roughage" or "bulk"), which includes cellulose, pectin, and other carbohydrates that the human body can digest poorly or not at all. Fiber is present in brown rice and whole wheat bread, but largely removed from white rice and white bread. All fruits and vegetables also contain varying amounts of fiber.*

*The government has not established an RDA for carbohydrate, but the amount of carbohydrate in a good diet can be derived as follows. Assume that a person needs 2500 calories daily obtained from fat, protein, and carbohydrate. Let us set the fat content of the diet at 36 percent of the calories—900 calories. (At 9 calories per gram, this implies 100 grams of fat, about 3½ ounces). The recommended 65 grams of protein provides 260 calories, at 4 calories per gram. The remaining 1340 calories must be obtained from carbohydrate. At 4 calories per gram, this amounts to 335 grams. Thus, a reasonable amount of carbohydrate to consume is 335 grams daily (about ¾ pound).

*Analytical methods for measuring the fiber content of foods are still primitive, so published values can be considered only approximations. "Crude fiber," the value for fiber reported in most scientific papers, is the amount meas-

The fiber content of the average diet may be dangerously low. This deficiency may be the chief cause of several illnesses of the digestive system and may be a secondary factor in other health problems. Fiber intake can be increased simply by eating more whole grain products, wheat bran, fruits, legumes, and vegetables.

Denis P. Burkitt, an eminent British surgeon, has been most prominent in gathering evidence on the importance of eating adequate amounts of fiber. Burkitt spent many years in service in rural African hospitals and became familiar with the health conditions of people whose diets were rich in dietary fiber. He noted that despite a heavy patient roster, there were almost no cases of appendicitis, constipation, or diverticular disease of the colon (a sometimes painful ailment that is common in the West). To verify his observations he sent questionnaires to a number of East African mission hospitals and received replies from twenty-five.[16] He also organized a medical safari to remote, rural hospitals to determine how many cases they recorded of each type of common "Western" disease. Finally, he conducted simple studies of the intestinal action of rural Africans, urban Africans, and Europeans living in Africa. Of these three groups, rural Africans consume the most fiber and the Europeans the least. His findings led him to conclude that some of the most common diseases of people who live on Western refined diets rarely afflict people who eat diets high in fiber and starch and low in sugar and fat.

---

ured by a harsh chemical (non-physiologic) method, which greatly underestimates the amount of fiber.

Burkitt and his colleagues believe that the increased consumption of refined flour (steel rollers for grinding flour were introduced in the 1880s) and the enormous rise in the consumption of sugar have contributed to the rise of degenerative diseases. Some of the diseases that Burkitt noticed were rare in rural Africa include varicose veins, obesity, deep venous thrombosis, intestinal polyps, bowel cancer, hiatal hernia, constipation, appendicitis, and diverticulosis.[17] There are interesting facts discussed below about the effects of fiber that might explain its relationship to some of these Western diseases, but it is premature to say that all these diseases are caused solely by a deficiency of dietary fiber. The rural African diet and life style differ from the Western diet and life style in more ways than just fiber content.

Persons on low-fiber Western diets have relatively small, hard, and infrequent stools. Such stools permit the colon to segment, which results in high pressures in the area of segmentation. The abnormally high pressures can cause outpouchings of the intestinal wall, i.e. painful diverticular disease or diverticulosis.[18] Thousands of Americans develop this serious, but unnecessary, disease every year. Gastroenterologists are now recommending that patients who suffer from diverticulosis, constipation, or irritable colon be treated with a high-fiber diet to soften the stool.[19] Adequate fiber produces a large, soft stool propelled without increased pressure and consequent risk of diverticulosis.

Drs. Heaton and Pomare of the University of Bristol in England, fed about one ounce of unprocessed wheat bran a day to fourteen subjects for a

44

period of up to two months; the results of the experiment showed a significant lowering of serum triglycerides[20] Triglycerides are a group of blood components that, when elevated, are associated with an increased risk of heart disease. Several studies also indicate that a high-fiber diet lowers blood cholesterol levels.[21, 22]

A diet high in fiber can help to prevent obesity, because high-bulk vegetable foods are comparatively low in calories. They also produce a full feeling that discourages overeating.

A number of medical writers and researchers, including Burkitt, have suggested that a deficiency of dietary fiber causes bowel cancer (cancer of the colon and rectum). However, there is little solid evidence to support this hypothesis. Population studies and laboratory experiments suggest that a diet high in fat is more closely linked to the development of bowel cancer, although fiber may be a secondary factor.[23]

As a prudent preventive measure, Americans should increase their consumption of dietary fiber. Fiber, because it occurs in fruits, whole grains, and vegetables, is associated with vitamins and minerals. Thus, diets rich in fiber are normally rich in many other nutrients, and for this reason alone, apart even from any effect in preventing the various diseases we have described, would be strongly recommended.

Foods receive two points per gram of fiber.

The third term of the carbohydrate factor—in addition to naturally occurring carbohydrates and fiber—is for the sugar (sucrose; cane or beet sugar), corn sugar (dextrose; glucose), and corn syrup that are added to food. Sugar is "pure food energy" or, in other words, "empty calories," because it does not contain vitamins, minerals, or protein. Sugar's empty calories will often squeeze nutritious foods out of the diet. Eating a lot of sugar may cause or aggravate tooth decay, obesity, heart disease, vitamin deficiencies, diabetes, and other health problems.

The average American—infant, adult, and golden-ager—consumes about 102 pounds of sugar a year; corn syrup, corn sugar, and other sweeteners add another 24 pounds.[25] The average person obtains almost 20 percent of his or her calories from sugar added to food. Some people consume much less sugar than the average, while others make sugar 25 percent or more of their diets. Americans have consumed tremendous amounts of sugar since the 1920s, according to USDA figures (see Figure 1). The 1972 level of 126 pounds of sugar and other sweeteners per person was 45 percent higher than in 1909 (87 pounds) and about three times as high as in the 1870s (40 pounds).[26] A major reason for the increase is the increasing availability of factory-made sweetened foods—candy, cakes, soda pop, ice cream, and certain breakfast cereals.

The price of sugar tripled in 1973-74. This economic force probably had the effect of more than a thousand warnings from the American Dental Association to help us reduce our intake of the harmless looking crystals. Sugar consumption dropped by 2 percent in 1974. (The sugar industry's soaring profits have prompted both the Department of Justice and the Council on Wage and Price Stability to investigate possible price fixing.)

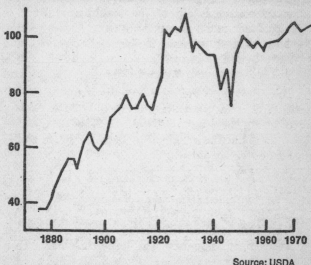

U.S. SUCROSE CONSUMPTION (per capita)

Source: USDA

Tooth decay (the technical name for which is "caries") is the most obvious of sugar's ill effects. Dr. B. Warren Ross, president of the American Society for Preventive Dentistry, reminds us that sugar's tooth-destroying ability is not a recent discovery. According to Ross:

The first recorded suggestion of a carbohydrate-caries relationship was made by Aristotle over two thousand years ago, when he wondered why soft and sweet figs produced damage to teeth. Since then other respected scientists like Galen, the Greek physician, and nu-

47

merous French, German, English, and Dutch investigators correlated sugar ingestion with poor dental health. The incidence of human caries in Europeans probably increased when sugar imports increased during the fifteenth century as a result of new trade routes to Europe from India and Arabia. Pierre Fauchard, the founder of dentistry as a profession, wrote in the eighteenth century: "All sugary food contributes not a little to the destruction of the teeth."[27]

Dr. Abraham Nizel, Associate Professor of Oral Health Services at Tufts University, told a Congressional Committee in March, 1973, what he had learned about the relationship between sugar and tooth decay. He said:

Over the last ten years, my students and I have done thousands of diet evaluations on patients with rampant caries at Tufts University School of Dental Medicine. We never found a single patient whose caries problem

> Tooth decay (caries) is avoidable: "In 1938, the diet of the natives of [Tristan da Cunha] consisted of two staples, potatoes and fish but no sugar. Not a single first permanent carious molar was found in any of the young people under the age of 20. In 1962, they were consuming an average of one pound of sugar per week, per person with the result that a comparable age group showed 50 percent of their molars to be carious." Dr. Abraham Nizel, School of Dental Medicine, Tufts University, 1973.

could not, in part, be traced to the patient's inordinate consumption of sugar. Every package of sugar-sweetened life savers, cough drops, breath mints, candies, chewing gum and soft drinks should be labeled with a statement warning that excessive frequent daily use of these products can produce significant amounts of dental plaque and dental decay.[28]

Dental researchers agree that sugar is most likely to lead to tooth decay when it is eaten in a solid or sticky form. A candy bar is much worse for the teeth than soda pop. Between-meal sugar is much more conducive to tooth decay than sugar eaten during a meal, because it is more likely to stick in the cracks and crevices of teeth. (Sugar itself does not cause decay; bacteria in the mouth digest the sugar and produce acid—it is this acid that eats away the teeth.)

The average American has five unfilled cavities. Army surveys show that every 100 inductees require 600 fillings, 112 extractions, 40 bridges, 21 crowns, 18 partial dentures, and one full denture! According to the Department of Agriculture, "It has been estimated that the incidence of dental caries in this country is progressing six times faster than the needed number of dentists can be trained."[29] According to the National Institute of Dental Research, America's annual dental bill would be an astonishing $13 billion if everyone got their teeth fully repaired.[30] As it is, we spend $5 billion a year on dental care, $2 billion of which goes toward repairing rotten teeth. The National Institute of Dental Research spends a measly $40,-000 a year on public information.

There is much debate in the nutrition community over sugar's contribution to heart disease. Dr. John Yudkin of London University (author of the book *Sweet and Dangerous*) and his followers argue that sugar is the major cause of heart disease, while some nutritionists pooh-pooh any connection whatsoever between sugar and heart disease. Studies of different populations have related high sugar consumption to high rates of heart disease, but the value of these studies is reduced because sugar and fat consumption often increase in tandem (much evidence has tied diets high in fat to heart disease). Several kinds of laboratory and human studies have related high-sugar diets to heart disease, and while the evidence is not conclusive, it is highly suggestive that sugar, in fact, is one of several factors that contribute to heart disease.

Surveys of individuals with and without heart disease have correlated the levels of triglycerides in the blood with the incidence of heart disease.[31] The level of triglycerides, in turn, partially reflects an individual's consumption of sugar.[32, 33] The National Institutes of Health recommends that people who have high blood levels of triglycerides eliminate sweets and desserts from their diets.

Some diseases are exacerbated by high-sugar diets, and increase the susceptibility of genetically prone individuals to heart disease. The most familiar of these is diabetes. Adult-onset diabetes may be aggravated by high levels of sugar consumption.[34] Diabetics experience a higher incidence of heart disease than the general population.[35]

The human love of sugar is undoubtedly natural, and is perhaps nature's way of encouraging us to eat sweet, nutritious fruit.[36] Every culture that has had the opportunity to eat sucrose-sweetened candy bars and drink soda pop has devoured such foods with great delight. The food industry has done everything possible to capitalize on the taste for sweet foods. Industry has sweetened foods that are not naturally sweet (like breakfast cereals), tempted children by describing in TV commericals how sweet and delicious their products are, and made sweet foods available wherever we turn. Industry cultivates a person's sweet tooth right from infancy. More than half of Gerber baby foods contain added sugar. The American baby starts off on sweetened baby food, graduates to sugar-coated breakfast cereals, and then to soda pop and cupcakes. Against all this encouragement to develop a sweet tooth and to eat sugary products, an occasional warning from a dentist, teacher, or parent is doomed to failure.

For sugars—sucrose, dextrose, and corn syrup—that are added to manufactured foods, we have deducted 2.5 points per gram per serving. Table 1 lists the sugar contents of many common foods.

Many natural foods contain sugars that are chemically identical to added sugars. However, we have not deducted points for naturally occurring sugar, because few persons consume excessive amounts of natural sugars and because most sugar-containing natural foods, such as fruits and milk, contain a wide variety of nutrients. Sugar is not a problem until refined sugar becomes an important part of a person's diet.

TABLE 1
Estimated Sugar Content of Food*

Food	Serving Size	Calories per Serving	Added Sugar as Percent of Total Weight**	Calories from Added Sugar as Percent of Total Calories
Hi-C orange drink	6 oz. (¾ c)	89	12	87
Cola	12 oz.	148	10	100
Bird's Eye Orange Plus	4 oz.	67	7	47
Bird's Eye Awake	4 oz.	51	11	94
Tang	4 oz.	61	13	93
Kool-Aid	8 oz.	98	11	98
Applesauce (sweetened)	1 cup	230	13	58
Del Monte canned peaches (water pack)	½ cup	38	0	0
Del Monte canned peaches (light syrup)	½ cup	73	7	48
Del Monte canned peaches (heavy syrup)	½ cup	101	12	61

Del Monte canned pineapple juice pack	½ cup	80	0	0
Del Monte canned pineapple (heavy syrup)	½ cup	105	5	24
Del Monte canned pineapple (extra heavy syrup)	½ cup	128	9	37
Del Monte fruit cup, diced peaches	5 oz.	107	13	65
Del Monte pudding cup, vanilla	5 oz.	190	18	50
Hunt-Wesson Snack Pack pudding	5 oz.	238	16	35
Hunt-Wesson Snack Pack fruit cup	5 oz.	96	9	49
Jello	½ cup	81	13	88
Duncan Hines angel food cake	1/12 cake	131	17	41
Duncan Hines blueberry muffin mix	1 muffin	39	12	38
Duncan Hines "Cake-like" brownies	1 brownie	152	50	30
Morton's coconut cream pie	¼ pie	273	24	33
Hostess Sno-Ball	1	159	42	50
Cracker Jack	1 box	150	68	66
Cool 'N Creamy	½ cup	203	8	20
Cool Whip	1 Tbsp.	16	24	26
M&M Plain	1 bag	210	—***	31

Food	Serving Size	Calories per Serving	Added Sugar as Percent of Total Weight**	Calories from Added Sugar as Percent of Total Calories
Milky Way	1 bar	240	—	30
Mars Almond	1 bar	215	—	24
Snickers	1 bar	240	—	24
3-Musketeers	1 bar	255	—	38
Hersheys milk chocolate	1 oz.	145	44	32
Sandwich cookie	⅜ oz.	50	35	27
White sugar	1 tsp.	16	100	100
	1 Tbsp.	40	100	100

*Calculations by the author; all companies refused to disclose the sugar contents of their products.
**Includes sugar (sucrose), corn sugar (dextrose), and corn syrup.
***Insufficient data.

Fat

$$\text{fat score} = \text{(fat quantity)}\ 0.2\ \text{(grams protein} + \text{grams carbohydrate} - 4\ \text{grams fat)} +$$

$$\text{(fat quality)}\ 0.5\ \text{(grams polyunsaturated} + \tfrac{1}{8}\ \text{grams oleic} - 4/3\ \text{grams saturated)}$$

The fat factor rates both the quantity and quality of the fat that is in a food. Fat is a necessary constitutent of the diet. It provides and facilitates the metabolism of fat-soluble vitamins (vitamins A, D, E, and K), contains the required nutrient linoleic acid, is an excellent source of energy, and provides bulk and flavor to meals. Too much calorie-rich fat, however, causes obesity and squeezes other nutrients out of the diet.

Many nutritionists recommend that fat provide no more than about one-third of one's calories, while a few recommend that fat contribute as little as 20 percent of one's calories. In 1909 fat contributed 32 percent of our calories. That figure is now up to 42 percent. Japanese, who enjoy a low incidence of heart disease (one-tenth the U.S. rate) and bowel cancer (one-fifth of the U.S. rate), consume a diet very low in fat.[37,38,39] Only 10 to 15 percent of their caloric intake comes from fat. As the Japanese are getting wealthier, however, they have begun to consume more meat and more fat. If this trend continues, Japanese medical schools had better begin training more cardiologists.

Our formula penalizes foods in which more than 36 percent of the calories come from fat. This amount of fat is equivalent to 20 percent of the food on a dry-weight basis. The maximum on this term is zero so that foods do not gain points simply for having little fat.

Several painless ways of reducing your fat intake (and possibly your waistline) include:

- Drinking skim milk (0 percent fat) or 2 percent milk (whole milk contains about 3.5 percent butterfat)
- Eating beans, grains, and cottage cheese instead of meat
- Not eating hot dogs or bologna—fat provides 80 percent of their calories
- Cutting off as much excess fat as possible from meat, both before and after you cook it
- Eating a different grade of meat. "Choice" and "prime" grade meat are high in fat; "good" grade cuts are low in fat, cheaper, and perfectly acceptable in stews, casseroles, etc.

That last point is worth expanding on. Meat grades—prime, choice, good—reflect the amount of fat marbling in the beef. The more fat marbling, the better the grade—and the higher the price. Although the higher-fat meat is reputed to have the best taste, a study by Consumers Union demonstrated that meat grade was a poor indicator of taste.[40] Also, certain varieties of cattle are said to be low in fat, but very flavorful. The current grading system is an incentive to the meat industry to raise cattle that is high in fat instead of being high in protein. The high-fat meat contributes to obesity, heart disease, and possibly other ailments. Also, the extra marbling is added by feeding cattle expensive grain in the feedlot. Not only does this increase the cost of meat, but it wastes tremendous amounts of grain. This grain could otherwise be sold to rich nations or donated to needy ones. Hopefully, the rising cost of feed grains and the recognition that wealthy nations have a moral obligation to assist poorer nations will persuade the Department of Agriculture to adopt a more enlightened grading system and the ranchers to employ more efficient ways of raising cattle.[41] Already, in fact, a few ranchers have turned to longhorn cattle and beefalo (a cross between buffalo and beef), which are low in fat, flavorful, and range-fed.

The kind of fat that is in a food is as important as the quantity. Eating too much saturated fat (which occurs primarily in animal fat, dairy products, hydrogenated vegetable oil,* and coconut

* Oils are liquid at room temperature; fats are solid at room temperature.

TABLE 2
Fat Content of Common Foods

Food	Percent of Calories from Fat	Saturated Fat	Oleic Acid*	Linoleic Acid**
			Percentage of Fat Calories from:	
Fruits, average	0			
Vegetables, average	0			
Milk, skim	0			
Cottage cheese, uncreamed	3			
Bread, whole wheat	11	22	43	22
Chicken, broiled	23	33	33	33
Sirloin steak, lean, broiled	40	45	45	—
Milk, 2% butterfat	31	54	27	—
Trout, raw	53	27	18	—
Ice cream (12% butterfat)	54	56	33	—
Eggs	63	35	43	9
Swiss cheese	68	54	32	4
Pork chop, cooked	73	38	43	10

Sirloin steak, lean and fat, broiled	74	45	45	—
Frankfurter, beef, cooked	80	45	45	—
Avocado (California)	90	18	47	12
Cream, whipping	96	53	30	3
Butter	100	57	33	2
Soybean oil	100	15	20	52
Margarine, regular	100	22	58	17
Margarine, made with liquid oil (varies according to brand)	100	23	38	36

Calculated from U.S. Department of Agriculture tables; all figures are approximate.

*A mono-unsaturated fat.

**The main polyunsaturated fat; the amounts of saturated fat, oleic acid, and linoleic acid do not add up to 100, because other mono-unsaturated and polyunsaturated fats are present.

oil) and too little polyunsaturated fat (which is abundant in vegetable oils) raises blood cholesterol levels and increases the risk of coronary heart disease, stroke, and other arterial diseases. Table 2 describes the fat content of some common foods, and Table 3 gives the percentage of fat in beef grades. These diseases killed about 900,000 Americans in 1970, far more than any other cause, and accounted for half of all deaths.[42] Heart disease is without doubt the number one health problem in the United States.

A cause and effect relationship between saturated fats and heart disease has not been proven beyond every doubt. However, many eminent researchers have concluded from studying a great body of scientific reasearch that eating too much saturated fat contributes to heart disease in many people, particularly men and older women.

Many studies have shown that the higher the level of cholesterol in blood, the greater the risk of

"In addition, virtually no steps have been taken by the food industry to reduce either the sugar content or the saturated fat and cholesterol content of foods. The technology of the food processing industry has made it possible to alter the fat and sugar content of a great variety of foods, but without public pressure few changes can be expected." Dr. Jean Mayer, Professor of Nutrition, Harvard School of Public Health, 1972.

TABLE 3

Typical Composition of the Average Beef Carcass*

GRADE	PROTEIN	FAT
Prime	14%	41%
Choice	15%	35%
Good	16.5%	28%

*Figures from U.S.D.A. Handbook No. 8.

heart disease. The most extensive and well-known of these studies was conducted in Framingham, Massachusetts. It and other studies have shown that the risk of coronary heart disease is five times as great for men 35-44 years of age who have cholesterol levels above 260 (milligrams per 100 milliliters of serum) as compared to men whose cholesterol levels are below 200.[43] Many studies have also shown that reducing the amount of saturated fat (and/or increasing the amount of polyunsaturated oil) in the diet reduces cholesterol levels. The National Diet-Heart Study, a two-year study involving test groups in six cities, showed that moderate changes in eating habits could reduce cholesterol levels by 14 percent.[44]

What has not been proven to the satisfaction of some researchers—a declining minority—is that eating more polyunsaturated fat and less saturated fat actually reduces the rate of heart disease. Studies bearing on this point are long, expensive, and difficult to control adequately. In one recent and impressive study, sponsored by the U.S. National Heart and Lung Institute, hundreds of patients in two mental hospitals in Finland were kept on special diets for six-year periods. For the first six-year period, patients in one hospital had a diet low in saturated fat and cholesterol and relatively high in polyunsaturated fat; patients in the other hospital had a diet that was relatively high in saturated fat and cholesterol and low in polyunsaturated fat. After six years, the diets in the two hospitals were switched. During both six-year periods blood cholesterol levels and the rate of deaths due to heart disease reflected the amount of saturated fat and cholesterol in the diets. The high saturated fat and cholesterol groups had a relatively high rate of fatal heart attacks.[45] Other studies, which were less carefully conducted, such as the New York Anti-Coronary Club experiment, have shown similar results.[46]

Although no perfect, large-scale diet-heart study has yet been conducted, most responsible health organizations urge Americans to consume what the American Heart Association calls a "prudent diet." This diet is low in fat and cholesterol and contains balanced amounts of saturated and polyunsaturated fats. The American Heart Association and the Inter-Society Commission for Heart Disease Resources both recommend that fat contribute no more than 35 percent of one's daily calorie intake and that saturated and polyunsaturated fat each contribute 10 percent or less of calories (most organizations and scientists warn against consuming too much polyunsaturated fat). The American Health Foundation, a private New York organization dedicated to preventing—rather than curing—disease, has adopted a "Position Statement on Diet and Coronary Heart Disease" that states:

The results do not unequivocally prove, but strongly suggest, that modification of diet with respect to type and amount of fat is effective in the prevention of coronary heart disease. There is no doubt that such modification is possible and that it is a feasible approach to controlling serum cholesterol. Furthermore, the evidence strongly suggests that diet modification can significantly reduce expected coronary heart disease morbidity [illness] and mortality [death]. . . .

In a joint statement in 1972, the American Medical Association and the Food and Nutrition Board of the National Academy of Sciences-National Research Council advised that:

There is extensive evidence that the level of cholesterol in the plasma of most people can be lowered by appropriate dietary modification. . . . Preliminary evidence suggests that faithful and continued consumption of a cholesterol-lowering diet over a period of years can reduce the coronary attack rate in middle-aged men. As would be expected in dealing with a chronic disease of this kind, early intervention appears to be more effective than intervention after the disease is evident.

The National Heart and Lung Institute (NHLI, a Federal government agency) in 1970 convened a Task Force of prestigious scientists to develop a long-range plan to combat arteriosclerosis. The next year the Task Force recommended that, among other things, NHLI should tell the public:

Current data indicate that the average North American has higher than optimal blood lipid [cholesterol, triglyceride] levels and ingests excessive calories, saturated fat, and cholesterol. Pending confirmation by appropriate diet or drug trials, it therefore would appear

63

prudent for the American people to follow a diet aimed at lowering serum lipid concentrations. For most individuals, this can be achieved by lowering intake of calories, cholesterol, and saturated fat.

Unfortunately, NHLI has not taken its Task Force's advice. NHLI remains the one important health organization that resists advising the American public (whose tax dollars pay for NHLI) to adopt a diet that is less conducive to heart disease. The current Director of NHLI, Dr. Robert Levy, an eminent researcher, told the author he is waiting for conclusive scientific proof that such a diet will reduce the incidence of heart disease. His desire to get to the bottom of things before speaking out would be highly commendable if he were working on an obscure scientific problem. However, while he waits, heart disease is killing hundreds of thousands of Americans a year, including about 165,000 people under the age of 65. One cannot help thinking that Levy fears that if his agency recommends a low-fat diet for the general public, the meat and dairy lobbies will force Congress to slash NHLI's budget. Scientists in USDA's Agricultural Research Service want their Department's educational branch to recommend a low-fat diet, but that branch will not budge until NHLI is willing to go along with the American Medical Association, American Heart Association, American Health Foundation, and all the other groups that have endorsed the moderate-fat diet.

In the past twenty-five years, our eating habits have changed considerably with respect to several foods that are thought to have a bearing on the influence of heart disease. Our consumption of vegetable fats, which are high in polyunsaturates, almost doubled between 1947-49 and 1973, going from 36 grams to 63 grams per day. In the same period, our consumption of relatively saturated fat of animal origin decreased from 105 to 93 grams per day.[47] Meanwhile, perhaps reflecting the American Heart Association's efforts and changes in our life style, per capita egg consumption dropped 24 percent between 1950 and 1972.[48] Eggs are a major source of cholesterol, which has been closely tied to heart disease. These dietary changes could be expected to lower the incidence of heart disease. In a report released by the National Center for Health Statistics in March, 1974, statisticians showed that the death rate for diseases of the heart has been dropping slowly and steadily for two decades. The age-adjusted death rate dropped a remarkable 15 percent between 1950 and 1969. Of course, we cannot prove what factors were responsible for this gratifying turnabout, but it is not unlikely that dietary changes made some contribution.

The Framingham and other studies have shown that factors other than dietary fat are "risk factors" in heart disease. Some of the other important factors are:

- Obesity
- Lack of exercise
- Genetic background (if all your ancestors died of heart disease, watch out)
- Cholesterol
- Cigarette smoking and air pollution
- High blood pressure

- Diabetes
- Anxiety
- Diets high in sugar

Thus, just using skim milk or a certain brand of margarine is no guarantee that you will not have a heart attack. If the epidemic of heart disease is to be reduced maximally in the United States, we will have to make several changes in our eating habits and life style. Our sedentary life style may be comfortable, convenient, and effortless in the short run, but deadly in the long run. Driving to work instead of bicycling or walking may be killing thousands of people a year. The countless automobiles that clog our city streets every day cause much more air pollution and anxiety than the small number of buses or subway trains that could replace them. The competitive, dog-eat-dog business world makes nervous wrecks of millions of us. Most of us can't afford the time or money it takes to get a proper medical examination that would tell us whether or not we are likely to develop heart disease. A modern society in which heart disease was not a major killer would be very different from present day America, but a goal well worth working toward.

In calculating the nutritional scores, foods are penalized two-thirds of a point per gram of saturated fat per serving, credited with one-half point per gram of polyunsaturated fat, and credited with one-sixth point per gram of mono-unsaturated fat. Mono-unsaturated fat has no apparent effect on blood cholesterol levels or the incidence of heart disease. If the fat in a food consists of equal amounts of the three kinds, the term is zero. Otherwise, the food gains or loses points, depending on the amounts of the different kinds of fat.

Table 4 rates fats and oils according to their content of linoleic acid, the major polyunsaturated oil.

TABLE 4

Comparison of Fats and Oils

FAT OR OIL	% LINOLEIC ACID*
Safflower	75
Sunflower	68
Corn	57
Cottonseed	54
Soybean	50
Sesame	43
Rice bran	32
Peanut	31
Olive	15
Lard	14
Cocoa butter	2
Butterfat	2
Coconut	2

*Linoleic acid is the major polyunsaturated oil.

You can increase the amount of polyunsaturated fat or reduce the amount of saturated fat in your diet by:

- Using margarines that contain "liquid oil" instead of regular margarine or butter
- Drinking skim milk or 2 percent milk instead

of whole milk
- Cooking food in vegetable oil instead of butter, margarine, or lard
- Not using cream in your coffee or tea (also avoid "coffee whiteners" that contain coconut oil, palm oil, or hydrogenated oil)
- Eating less meat and cutting off the fat from the meat you do eat
- Eating fruit for dessert instead of ice cream

Vitamins and Minerals

$$\text{vitamin and} \atop \text{mineral score} = \frac{\text{milligrams of each vitamin or mineral/serving}}{\text{RDA of each vitamin or mineral}} \times 50$$

Vitamins and minerals are two essential kinds of chemicals that we obtain from food. Most vitamins and minerals work closely with specific proteins to enable the body to obtain energy from food, build new tissue, and synthesize needed chemicals. Vitamins and minerals cannot be produced by the body* and must be obtained from food. The

*Either the body or bacteria in the large intestine can produce some vitamins, but the amounts are usually too small to allow optimal growth of the individual.

amount of these nutrients in a food may vary significantly, depending on the climatic conditions in which a plant grew, the food an animal ate, the way the food was processed, and the time at which a vegetable or fruit was picked. Tomatoes that are exposed to the sun while growing have more vitamin C than tomatoes shaded by leaves. Carrots develop more vitamin A as they mature, so fresh carrots may have less vitamin A than canned carrots. which are picked at later stages of maturity.

A person's need for vitamins and minerals depends to some extent on the composition of his or her diet. For instance, a diet high in sugar and starch leads to an increased demand for thiamin (vitamin B-1). A diet that is excessively high in protein can lead to a pyridoxine (vitamin B-6) deficiency, and this deficiency can in turn reduce the absorption of vitamin B-12 from food. The interrelationships between vitamins, minerals, and the rest of the diet are many, complex, and still not entirely understood by nutrition researchers.

"Some of the differences in the concentration of nutrients in plants that result from variations in the environment or varieties may appear small. A small increase in the amount of a vitamin, mineral, or other essential nutrient, however, may mean the difference between an adequate or inadequate level of that nutrient in a diet." U.S. Dept. of Agric., 1959 Yearbook.

Drugs, too, can influence the body's nutritional needs. The birth control pill increases a woman's requirement for vitamin B-6, and is now (belatedly) being studied for other subtle effects. To be on the safe side, women on the pill, and people taking other drugs, should ask their doctor about taking a vitamin-mineral supplement.

An individual's genetic make-up can also influence his or her need for selected vitamins and minerals. Dr. Roger J. Williams, the University of Texas biochemist who discovered one of the B vitamins, has written extensively on wide variations in nutritional needs from one person to another. Williams' fascinating little book, *Biochemical Individuality*, is well worth reading.

A person's nutrient requirements are relatively independent of one's caloric needs. In other words, a person would need approximately the same amounts of the various nutrients whether one led a rather sedentary life as an artist or a more active daily routine as, say, a hiking guide. Calorie needs would differ greatly, but not nutrient needs. Thus, active people who eat a varied diet containing 3000 calories might easily consume enough of each nutrient, but if they changed their life style so as to need only 1500 calories a day, they might simply not eat enough food to obtain adequate amounts of all the necessary nutrients. Many people not only consume low-calorie diets, but many of those calories are pure sugar and fat and are not associated with any significant amounts of vitamins, minerals, protein, or fiber. Persons whose diet is one-fifth soda pop, chewing gum, and candy must obtain

100 percent of their nutrients from only 80 percent of their food.

For our rating system, the amount of vitamin A, thiamin (or pyridoxine), riboflavin, niacin, ascorbic acid, iron, and calcium (or magnesium) in a serving of food is divided by its RDA and multiplied by a coefficient of 50. A serving of food that contained 100 percent of the RDA of a vitamin or mineral would receive 50 points. The upper limit is 50 for each nutrient.

In the following pages, we discuss the importance and interesting features of these vitamins and minerals that help determine a food's rating. Many other vitamins and minerals are as important for good health as the ones discussed here. They are not included in the formula primarily because the amounts present in commercially available foods have too seldom been determined by manufacturers or the government.

VITAMIN A

If people were quizzed on their knowledge of nutrition, vitamin A would surely be one of the best known nutrients. Most people know that severe deficiencies of vitamin A can cause poor vision or even blindness. Less well known is the vital contribution this vitamin makes to the development of teeth and the health of mucous membranes and skin. Healthy mucous membranes form a vital link in the body's defenses against infection. Severe vitamin A deficiency leads to "dry eye" (xerophthalmia), which is a major and tragic cause of blindness in the Orient. There the problem is not so much a shortage of the vitamin as an ignorance of the necessity to eat foods rich in it.

In America, the Ten-State Nutrition Survey revealed that many persons consume far less than the recommended amount of vitamin A. Many of these persons may have "night blindness," which is the eye's inability to readjust rapidly after being struck by bright light. Night blindness can be a real highway hazard. Eating a rich source of vitamin A can cure night blindness in short order.

Vitamin A occurs in liver, eggs, and dairy products. Many breakfast cereals are fortified with this vitamin. Carotene, a substance that the body converts to vitamin A, occurs in collard greens, broccoli, carrots, sweet potatoes, watermelon, spinach, and many other vegetables and fruits. The availability of and necessity for vitamin A, like other vitamins, depends on the person, the food, and the diet. Fat and protein both increase the absorption of the vitamin from the intestinal tract. Scoreboard 2 lists many of the best sources of vitamin A (fortified breakfast cereals are not included in this and subsequent Scoreboards; read the label to find out how much vitamin A and other nutrients were added to such cereals).

Vitamin A is one of the few vitamins that the body stores. A person can manage without any new vitamin A for many weeks, if his or her reserves have been built up. However, if that person's diet is very low in protein (not a problem in the United States), the vitamin cannot be released from the liver into the bloodstream. Because vitamin A is stored in the liver, that organ is one of the best dietary sources. One serving of liver can easily supply a week's worth of vitamin A.

While too little vitamin A is a problem for many people who cannot afford vitamin-rich food or whose meals do not include sources of vitamin A, occasional problems of too much vitamin A arise. Symptoms of excesses include fatigue, severe headaches, insomnia, and loss of body hair. Because high-potency vitamin capsules offer the greatest opportunity for overdoses, the Federal government recently restricted the dosage of vitamin A capsules.

SCOREBOARD 2
Foods Rich in Vitamin A
(the average person needs 50 points per day)

Food	Serving Size	Vitamin A Score*
Collard greens, frozen	3⅓ oz.	50
Broccoli spears, frozen	3⅓ oz.	50
Turnip greens	3⅓ oz.	50
Sweet potato, baked	3⅓ oz.	50
Liver, beef or chicken	2 oz.	50
Spinach	3⅓ oz.	50
Cantaloupe	¼ melon	49
Watermelon	2 pounds**	25
Tomato	1	16
V-8 juice	4 oz.	14

Food	Serving Size	Vitamin A Score*
Peach	1	13
Eggs	2	12

*Double these numbers to determine the percentage of RDA for vitamin A that a food contributes to the diet.

**This average-sized serving includes the rind; however, nutrients in the rind were not included in the score.

THIAMIN

All of the B-vitamins are characterized by their ability to dissolve in water and thiamin (vitamin B-1) is no exception. In addition, thiamin is relatively unstable. It is easily destroyed by heat, so pork, peas, wheat germ, nuts, beans, and other rich sources of the vitamin should not be overcooked (but be sure not to undercook pork or you may encounter the nasty trichina worm). Thiamin and its B-vitamin cousins are crucial components of enzymes.

SCOREBOARD 3

Good Sources of Thiamin
(the average person needs 50 points per day)

Food	Serving Size	Thiamin Score*
Yeast, brewer's	1 Tbsp.	42
Pork chop, lean	1.7 oz.	18

Food	Serving Size	Thiamin Score*
Pork sausage	2 links	14
Roast ham, lean and fat**	3 oz.	13
Rye bread	2 slices	10
Green peas, frozen	½ cup	10
White bread, enriched	2 slices	8
Wheat germ	2 Tbsp.	8
Spam**	2 oz.	7
Bacon**	3 slices	7
Pork and beans	½ cup	7
Peas and carrots, frozen	½ cup	7
Whole wheat bread	2 slices	6
Spaghetti, macaroni, egg noodles, enriched	¾ cup (1 oz. dry)	6
Oatmeal	1 cup	6
Heinz Great American Split Pea and Smoked Ham soup**	1 cup	6
Asparagus, frozen	3⅛ oz.	6
Beef liver	2 oz.	5
Cashew nuts	¼ cup	5

*Double these numbers to determine the percentage of RDA for thiamin that a food contributes to the diet.

**These foods contain sodium nitrite, an additive that should be avoided.

A diet rich in carbohydrate increases the body's need for thiamin; when that carbohydrate is sugar the need is increased even further.[49] People who try to survive on soda pop and potato chips may not obtain enough of this vitamin. So if you need any extra excuses to throw away that bottle of Coke, here's a good one.

Thiamin is essential for a properly functioning nervous system. A severe deficiency of the vitamin can lead to the illnesses known as beriberi and Wernicke's syndrome. It is possible that less severe deficiencies cause milder mental problems. Because Wernicke's syndrome was particularly common among alcoholics, public health officials once contemplated requiring distillers to add thiamin to booze.

In 1965 the average American consumed about 1.8 milligrams of thiamin a day. This amount is sufficient to prevent beriberi. Five hundred years ago, despite a lack of fortified breakfast cereals and enriched bread, English peasants were consuming about two-and-one-half times as much (4.2 milligrams)![50]

RIBOFLAVIN

One of the reasons milk and foods containing milk are so nutritious is that they contain generous amounts of riboflavin (vitamin B-2). In fact, most Americans get almost half of their riboflavin from milk, cheese, and other diary products. One benefit that the disappearance of the milkman has had is that we are probably getting a little more of this vitamin than we used to (assuming we drink about the same amount of milk). Riboflavin is rapidly destroyed by light, and when glass bottles of milk sat on our sunlit doorsteps much of the riboflavin in milk was destroyed—as much as 10 percent in thirty minutes and 40 percent in two hours. Paper cartons or dark glass protect the vitamin. (Whether the unemployed milkmen and their families are getting enough riboflavin is another story.) Liver, meat, fortified breakfast cereals, and whole and enriched grain products are other rich sources of riboflavin.

SCOREBOARD 4

Riboflavin Sources
(the average person needs 50 points per day)

Food	Serving Size	Riboflavin Score*
Beef liver	2 oz.	50
Chicken liver	2 oz.	45
Liver sausage**	2 oz.	27
Buttermilk	8 oz.	13
Yogurt	8 oz.	13
Swanson deep dish beef meat pie	16 oz.	13
Milk, whole	8 oz.	12
Yeast, brewer's	1 Tbsp.	10
Almonds	¼ cup	10
Avocado	½	9
Cottage cheese, creamed	½ cup	9
Cottage cheese, uncreamed	½ cup	8
Cheddar cheese	2 oz.	8
Leg of lamb, lean and fat, roasted	3 oz.	7
American cheese	2 oz.	7
		77

Food	Serving Size	Riboflavin Score*
Swiss cheese	2 oz.	6
Veal cutlet	3 oz.	6
Leg of lamb, lean	2½ oz.	6
Hamburger, lean	3 oz.	6
Rye bread	2 slices	6
Turnip greens	3⅞ oz.	6
White bread, enriched	2 slices	6
Lamb chop, lean	2.6 oz.	6

*Double these numbers to determine the percentage of RDA for riboflavin that a food contributes to the diet.

**This food contains sodium nitrite, an additive that should be avoided.

"Nutritional surveys reported out in both the U.S. and Canada within the last five years have demonstrated an embarrassing number of people in both countries with measurable malnutrition of one kind or another, particularly relating to certain vitamins or minerals. I say embarrassing because we have the knowledge and other kinds of resources necessary to prevent this kind of disorder, and yet even a conservative estimate of the number of cases in the United States would get into the millions." Dr. Virgil Wodicka, Director, FDA Bureau of Foods, 1974.

Some of the first symptoms of riboflavin deficiency are cracks at the sides of the mouth and a soreness and redness of the tongue and lips: the little papillae on the tongue decline in size. Severe riboflavin deficiency is a rarity in the United States, although much of the population consumes less than the recommended amount.

NIACIN

Niacin, sometimes called vitamin B-3, helps living cells generate energy. Niacin deficiency—pellagra—leads to skin eruptions, an inflamed mucous membrane which causes the tongue and mouth to swell and become sore, diarrhea, and irritation of the rectum. Persons often experience irritability and depression, and in advanced cases of pellagra, delirium, hallucinations, and stupor occur. Pellagra is prevalent among people who have a monotonous diet high in corn and was widespread in the southern United States until public health officials ordered corn meal to be fortified with niacin.

Niacin occurs in many foods, particularly chicken (light meat contains 50 percent more niacin than dark meat), liver, tuna and salmon, red meat, and peanuts. In addition, the body can manufacture niacin from tryptophan, one of the amino acids in protein. (Corn-rich diets lead to pellagra largely because corn protein contains very little tryptophan and because the niacin is not readily available.) That niacin can be obtained in two ways greatly complicated the early investigations into the cause of pellagra.

SCOREBOARD 5
Good Sources of Niacin
(the average person needs 50 points per day)

Food	Serving Size	Niacin Score*
Chicken, breast	3 oz.	31
Tuna, packed in oil	3 oz.	25
Beef liver	2 oz.	23
Chicken liver	2 oz.	17
Turkey meat	3 oz.	16
Peanuts	¼ cup	15
Sockeye salmon, canned	3 oz.	15
Hamburger, lean	3 oz.	12
Round steak, lean and fat	3 oz.	12
Leg of lamb, lean and fat	3 oz.	12
Veal cutlet	3 oz.	11
Lamb chop, lean	2½ oz.	11
Bounty chicken stew	1 cup	11
Leg of lamb, lean	2½ oz.	11
Sirloin steak	3 oz.	10
Lamb chop, lean and fat	3 oz.	10
Pot roast	3 oz.	9
Campbell Chunky Chicken soup	1 cup	8
Roast ham**	3 oz.	8
Yeast, brewer's	1 Tbsp.	7
Cod, broiled	3 oz.	7

*Double these numbers to determine the percentage of RDA for niacin that a food contributes to the diet.
**This food contains sodium nitrite, an additive that should be avoided.

The best known vitamin of all is vitamin C, or ascorbic acid—and it is also one of the most unusual. A vitamin, by definition, is a chemical that an animal needs for growth and development, but of which the animal cannot itself produce adequate quantities. The animal must obtain the chemical from its food. Millions of years ago man's early ancestors lost the ability to produce ascorbic acid. From then on, gorillas, monkeys, and man were fated to require ascorbic acid in their diets— or suffer a disorder called scurvy. The inability to produce ascorbic acid can be considered a genetic defect that all primates (and the guinea pig, bulbul bird, and Indian fruit-eating bat) share. Elephants, chipmunks, dogs, and other animals can produce ascorbic acid within their own tissues and never have to worry about scurvy. For them, ascorbic acid is not a vitamin.

Occasional cases of vitamin C deficiency in infants have been observed, due primarily to poor feeding practices. The baby's bones do not develop properly and its joints are swollen and tender. In adults, signs of scurvy are most obvious in soft tissue. Gums become sore, swollen, and may bleed and get infected readily. Blood vessels weaken and may rupture, sometimes leading to anemia. The healing of wounds is severely impaired.

Amazingly, despite the year-round availability of foods that contain vitamin C, several Americans have died of severe scurvy in recent years. These persons were adhering to a Zen macrobiotic diet. In the most extreme form of this diet, followers consume only brown rice and water. Brown rice is an excellent food, but it contains absolutely no vitamin C. One woman adamantly refused a doctor's advice to take vitamin C, proclaiming her faith in the healing powers of the all-rice diet until the angels carried her away. Extremes in eating invite trouble.[51]

The vitamin C content of a fruit depends in large part upon how much sun it receives. A peach in the middle of a tree, a tomato growing in the shade of a leaf, or turnips growing in a cloudy, rainy year, will have relatively little vitamin C. Some varieties of apples (such as Northern Spy, Gravenstein, and Willowtwig) have two or three times as much vitamin C as other varieties (McIntosh and Rome Beauty).

Some of the best dietary sources of vitamin C are listed in Scoreboard 6.

In recent years, largely through the persistent efforts of Linus Pauling, Professor of Chemistry at Stanford University, many persons in and out of the medical profession now believe that human health might be significantly improved if we consumed amounts of vitamin C much larger than can be obtained conveniently from food.[52] The recommended intake of the vitamin for adults is about 60 milligrams per day, but most animals synthesize a much larger amount (in proportion to their weight). Several studies* have indicated that high

*These were "double-blind" studies, designed to minimize biases and psychosomatic effects.

doses (1 gram per day) of vitamin C can reduce the frequency and/or severity of the common cold, but the most recent and carefully controlled studies have shown only a minor effect or no effect at all.[53] On balance, the evidence seems to indicate that vitamin C has a mild beneficial effect with regard to colds. However, much research is needed to determine whether the massive doses are hazardous to the general public or to particular segments of the population. Dr. Victor Herbert, Clinical Professor of Pathology and Medicine at Columbia University, has found that large doses of vitamin C can destroy 50 to 95 percent or more of the vitamin B-12 in a meal.[54] Also, the abrupt withdrawal of a high daily dose can cause abnormally low blood levels of ascorbic acid. Dr. T. W. Anderson, Professor of Epidemiology and Biometrics at the University of Toronto, has conducted several recent studies on vitamin C and the common cold. He concluded one paper with these words of advice:

In view of these potential hazards, and in the absence of any evidence that the higher intakes are associated with any additional benefits, it would seem prudent to advise the public against the regular daily ingestion of doses of vitamin C of 1 gram or more. However, the possibility remains that a modest supplementation of some diets may be desirable, and that short-term heroic doses of vitamin C may prove to be justified during acute infection and possibly other forms of stress.[51]

SCOREBOARD 6

Good Sources of Vitamin C
(the average person needs 50 points per day)

Food	Serving Size	Vitamin C Score*
Orange	1	50
Orange juice, fresh or frozen	4 oz.	50
Hi-C orange drink (fortified)	6 oz.	50
Brussel sprouts	½ cup	50
Broccoli, frozen	3⅓ oz.	50
Collard greens	3⅓ oz.	50
Del Monte fruit cup (fortified)	5 oz.	50
Hunt's tomato paste	½ cup	50
Tang (fortified)	4 oz.	50
Broccoli, frozen, chopped	3⅓ oz.	42
Cauliflower, frozen	3⅓ oz.	42
Strawberries	½ cup	40
Cantaloupe	¼ melon	39
Turnip greens	3⅓ oz.	37
Grapefruit	½	37
Cabbage, raw, chopped	1 cup	35
Tomato	1	35
Awake (fortified)	4 oz.	32
Orange Plus (fortified)	4 oz.	30
Spinach, frozen	3⅓ oz.	30
Hunt's tomato sauce	½ cup	27
Watermelon	2 pounds**	25
Tangerine	1	22

Food	Serving Size	Vitamin C Score*
Pineapple, raw, diced	1 cup	20
Asparagus, frozen	3⅓ oz.	20
V-8 juice	4 oz.	18
Avocado, Florida	½	18
Spinach, frozen, chopped	3⅓ oz.	18
Sweet potato, baked	3⅓ oz.	17
Potato, baked	3⅓ oz.	16
Tomato juice	4 oz.	16
Campbell tomato soup	1 cup	14

*Double these numbers to determine the percentage of RDA for vitamin C that a food contributes to the diet.
**The weight includes the rind; however, any nutrients in the rind were not included in the score.

IRON

America is the richest and one of the best-fed nations in the world, yet many of us suffer from iron deficiency. Iron is vital to good health, because it enables red blood cells to carry oxygen from our lungs to all parts of our body. Infants and pregnant and lactating (nursing) women are especially likely to be deficient (anemic), and require iron tablets or iron-fortified foods. The preliminary findings of the First Health and Nutrition Examination Survey (HANES), which was conducted by the Department of Health, Education and Welfare, showed that the average 18- 44-year-old woman was consuming only 58 percent of the recommended intake of iron. Only 7 percent of the women consumed the recommended amount (18 milligrams).

You may wonder how people in less affluent countries and earlier eras managed to survive and flourish without the help of Geritol and iron-fortified cereal products. Well, first, many people outside of the United States do *not* receive enough iron from their food. But another answer is that many people eat and ate better than we do. For example, Sir Jack Cecil Drummond, an English food historian and Professor of Biochemistry, has calculated that the diet of a 15th century peasant contained 21 milligrams of iron a day.[50] That compares with the 16.5 milligrams that the average American consumed in 1965 in the form of natural and fortified foods. The peasants certainly ate more food and less junk foods. Good sources of iron are listed in Scoreboard 7.

SCOREBOARD 7

Good Sources of Iron
(the average person needs 50 points per day)

Food	Serving Size	Iron Score*
Liver, chicken or beef	2 oz.	14
Chili con carne with beans	1 cup	12
Blackstrap molasses	1 Tbsp.	9

Food	Serving Size	Iron Score*
Round steak	3 oz.	8
Pot roast	3 oz.	8
Hamburger	3 oz.	8
Campbell chili beef soup	1 cup	8
Lima beans	½ cup	8
Veal cutlet	3 oz.	7
Navy beans	½ cup	7
Soy beans	½ cup	7
Pork and beans	½ cup	7
Campbell Chunky Beef soup	1 cup	7
Sirloin steak	3 oz.	7

*Double these numbers to determine the percentage of RDA for iron that a food contributes to the diet.

An interesting thing about iron is that the body absorbs it from food at widely ranging rates. The exact amount of iron that is absorbed from a food depends on the composition of the meal and on the eater's previous intake of iron. For instance, a well-nourished body will absorb only about 5 to 10 percent of the iron in the diet. But when a body is deficient in iron it absorbs 15 to 20 percent of the iron. The nature of the food in which iron occurs is also an important factor in absorption. Iron is absorbed better from meat than from eggs and green vegetables. Beans contain a great deal of iron, but it is not nearly so well absorbed as the iron in meat. However, if the beans are eaten with meat, the iron in the beans will be absorbed better. Ascorbic acid (vitamin C) and other acids enhance the absorption of iron.

CALCIUM

Children—whose bones are growing rapidly—need lots of milk, because that is one of the few good sources of calcium. Vitamin D, which is often added to milk, plays an essential role in enabling the body to absorb this important mineral. When relatively little calcium is present in a person's diet, the body absorbs it more efficiently. Anxiety may reduce the rate of absorption. Some calcium-rich foods are listed in Scoreboard 8.

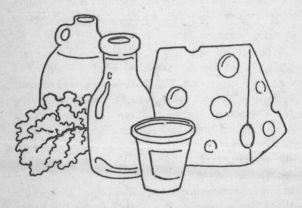

Some vegetables contain calcium, but in a form that is not as available as the calcium in milk. Wheat contains phytic acid, and spinach, chard, and rhubarb contain oxalic acid. (Collards, turnip and mustard greens, and kale are high in calcium and contain little oxalic acid.) Both phytic and oxalic acids can bind calcium and reduce its availability to the body, however this has not been known to cause calcium deficiencies in Americans. A problem would arise only if most of one's calcium comes from certain vegetable foods and if one is deficient in vitamin D, a rare combination in the United States. (Vitamin D is added to milk and occurs naturally in fish liver oil; in the presence of sunlight, our skin tissue converts cholesterol to vitamin D.) The combination of too little sunshine, too little vitamin D, and poorly absorbable calcium causes adult rickets or osteomalacia.

SCOREBOARD 8

Good Sources of Calcium
(the average person needs 50 points per day)

FOOD	SERVING SIZE	CALCIUM SCORE*
Swiss cheese	2 oz.	25
Cheddar cheese	2 oz.	21
American cheese	2 oz.	20
Milk, skim or whole	8 oz.	15
Yogurt	8 oz.	15
Sockeye salmon, canned	3 oz.	11
Collard greens	3⅓ oz.	9
Turnip greens	3⅓ oz.	8
New England clam chowder	8 oz.	8

Food	Serving Size	Calcium Score*
Blackstrap molasses	1 Tbsp.	7
Kale, with stems	3⅓ oz.	6
Franco-American macaroni and cheese	1 cup	6
Cottage cheese, creamed	½ cup	6

*Double these numbers to determine the percentage of RDA for calcium that a food contributes to the diet.

Refined grain products (white bread, spaghetti, rice) and breakfast cereals are often "enriched" or "fortified" with some or all of the two minerals and five vitamins discussed above. The refining process, however, removes many other important nutrients that are not replaced. So that these foods are not unduly rewarded for having a few selected nutrients, their ratings are calculated by replacing thiamin by pyridoxine (vitamin B-6), and calcium by magnesium. Even with this adjustment, some heavily fortified foods are little more than starchy vitamin pills and may have scores higher than their overall nutritional values merit. Many ready-to-eat breakfast cereals and beverages fall into this category.

MAGNESIUM

Magnesium plays an extremely important role in human metabolism. The mineral is part of many enzymes and plays a unique role in muscle contraction. Magnesium occurs in virtually all foods, but is especially abundant in nuts, peanuts, beans, whole grains, blackstrap molasses, and dairy products.

Despite the widespread occurrence of magnesium in foods, some Americans may be suffering deficiencies. According to the Department of Agriculture, in the early years of this century, the average American ingested about 410 milligrams of magnesium a day. In 1965 that figure was down to 340 milligrams. The recommended daily intake is 400 milligrams. Dr. D. Mark Hegsted, Professor of Nutrition at Harvard University, believes that "magnesium deficiency may be a substantial clinical problem."[55] Animals that are fed diets low in magnesium are highly susceptible to arterial diseases. Dr. Roger Williams wrote that "mild magnesium deficiency may be widespread, and a disastrous deficiency may not be uncommon among those suffering from heart attacks."[56] Williams has pointed out that magnesium deficiency in animals leads to extreme nervousness—whether mild deficiencies in people have a similar effect is not known.

When whole wheat flour is refined to white flour, the outer, magnesium-rich layers of the wheat berry are removed. Approximately 85 percent of the magnesium is lost. None of this valuable nutrient is restored when bread is enriched. Many breakfast cereals are fortified with magnesium.

Pyridoxine (vitamin B-6) is a crucial component of the enzymes in the body that produce amino acids (which the body uses to make protein) and that metabolize carbohydrate. A deficiency of this vitamin reduces the formation of antibodies, which are made of protein, and thus may decrease the body's resistance to disease.

Pyridoxine can be destroyed by heat and should be replaced in heat-processed foods. In the early 1950s, infants became ill when the pyridoxine in their milk formula was destroyed by heat processing. The babies became irritable and developed muscular twitching and convulsive seizures.

The body's need for pyridoxine is increased by a diet high in sugar or protein—the typical American diet. A woman's need is increased further by oral contraceptives.[57] Good sources of pyridoxine are meat, liver, vegetables, and whole grains. As with many other nutrients, pyridoxine is lost when whole grains are refined. The amount that is lost when wheat is refined—thirty-two billion milligrams a year—would supply the average eater with 15 percent of his or her recommended daily allowance. This vitamin is not replaced in enriched bread, but is added to many fortified breakfast foods.

"Life is a delicate balance of a seemingly infinite number of competing chemical and physiological processes. The trace elements are obviously of great importance to these processes and to that balance." This is what the U.S. Department of Agriculture concluded about trace elements in its 1959 Yearbook.

The body needs only tiny, or *trace*, amounts of zinc, copper, manganese, chromium, molybdenum, and certain other minerals, but they are absolutely essential for good health. Most of these elements occur in many foods, so people who eat a balanced diet should not have deficiencies. However, according to Dr. Leon Hopkins, a trace mineral specialist at the Department of Agriculture's Fort Collins, Colorado, laboratory:

Trace element deficiencies do exist in large numbers of people in this country. . . . We can not assume that animals, including man, are obtaining adequate amounts of the various trace elements for optimum health from plant foods. Soil depletion, increased processing of foods and feeds, and changing eating patterns are forcing us to change our concepts in mineral nutrition.[58]

Traditionally, the sign of a vitamin or mineral deficiency was an obvious physical impairment. Doctors looked for scurvy, rickets, stunted growth, goiter, etc. It was assumed that if a person did not have any of these overt symptoms he or she consumed an adequate amount of vitamins, minerals, and trace elements. In recent years, however, scientists have begun studying more subtle effects of marginal, but prolonged, deficiencies of trace minerals. These deficiencies may cause diseases that take many years to develop, such as heart disease, or cause such problems as slow healing of wounds, lower resistance to diseases, and decreased absorption or utilization of nutrients. These deficiencies would have a much greater impact on elderly and infirm people than on the healthy.

Dr. Henry Schroeder of Dartmouth University, one of the trail-blazers in this field, has pointed out that livestock and laboratory animals are fed considerably more trace minerals than man receives. Farmers and scientists both know how important these substances are for optimum growth and health.

Trace minerals are present in natural foods, but certain food processing practices and the priorities of the food industry have led to a precarious situation for many Americans. Refined sugar and flour, which constitute about 40 percent of our diet, do not contribute their share of trace elements. Minerals are concentrated in the germ and bran of the

"There is merit also to the suggestion of Roberts that attempts be made through school boards to place a zone around school buildings in which the sale of candy and soft drinks would be prohibited." Council on Foods and Nutrition, American Medical Association, 1942.

wheat grain, and these are the very parts that are removed when grain is processed into white flour. None of the trace elements are restored to "enriched" flour or bread. Furthermore, the food industry and our own laziness are leading us to consume more and more convenience and snack foods that are composed of oil, water, refined flour, and sugar—high in calories, low in trace minerals and other nutrients. Dr. Schroeder wrote that, "The average American diet . . . is probably marginal, and in some cases, partly deficient in several essential micro-nutrients, especially . . . chromium, zinc, and possibly manganese."

Dr. K. Michael Hambidge, Assistant Professor of Pediatrics at the University of Colorado Medical Center, recently discovered children in Denver who had zinc deficiency. These were not starving, ghetto-dwelling, black children—they were all apparently healthy children from upper- or middle-class families. Zinc is a necessary part of many enzymes, and moderate deficiencies could possibly impair one's health. Most of the children with zinc deficiency were smaller and lighter than other children their age. Dr. Hambidge and his colleagues also found that the children had an abnormally poor sense of taste, a phenomenon that has been tied to zinc deficiency.[60]

An area that is receiving an increasing amount of attention is the possible relationship between the mineral content of drinking water and risk of heart disease. In general, the lower the mineral content (that is, the softer the water), the greater the incidence of heart disease in that community. One exception to this rule seems to be in the Midwest, where Kansas City, Kansas, has a 50 percent higher incidence of heart disease than Kansas City, Missouri, although the Missouri water is softened. The exception may be due to the fact that Kansans' blood contains ten times as much cadmium and one-third as much zinc as the blood of their neighbors across the river.[61]

The moral of the story—if you can bear hearing it again—is to eat whole grain products, nuts and vegetables; sprinkle wheat germ on your foods; and avoid sugar and white bread.

The following foods are rich in trace minerals and receive 2.5 points per ounce: shellfish, whole grains, liver, kidney, beans, peanuts, tree nuts.

III. What the Formula Does not Cover

THE FORMULA THAT we use to rate the nutritive values of foods has inherent limitations. First, it considers only a limited number of vitamins and minerals. Perforce, it was possible to include only those for which information is available for most foods. This prevented the inclusion of pantothenic acid, zinc, folic acid, and other essential nutrients.

The formula also leaves out other factors that are important considerations when we buy food, but that do not lend themselves to being part of a formula. In this section, we discuss briefly some of the topics not included in the formula.

Food Additives

The periodic discovery that a chemical widely used in our food may be dangerous has made millions of Americans extremely cautious about all food additives. In the last few years, cyclamate, DEPC (a preservative), and Violet No. 1 dye (the coloring used to stamp USDA's insignia on inspected meat) have been banned, and several others have come under suspicion. Most food additives are safe and some are positively beneficial. However, a few are hazardous, and some of the safe ones may be used to cheat or deceive shoppers— these are the additives that spark concern. If a widely used additive proves to be hazardous, thousands or even millions of people may be harmed.

Dr. Jacqueline Verrett, one of two brave scientists at FDA who revealed to the American public the problems with the artificial sweetener cyclamate, described the woefully inadequate job that FDA is doing in a recent book entitled *Eating May Be Hazardous to Your Health.* She wrote, "Notwithstanding the FDA's proclamations to the contrary, all is not right with our food supply and we had best do something about it ... our food supply is permeated with chemicals of dubious safety."

Nutrients are used as additives in enriched bread, milk, some breakfast cereals, and a few other products. These added nutrients are given full credit in our calculations. The rating system, however, does not deduct credit for food additives that are potentially harmful or that are used to deceive the consumer. It is impossible to assign values to these additives—foods containing them should simply not be eaten.

Artificial colors are usually used in food to replace real fruit or other natural products. Strawberry soda pop, for instance, never contains natural coloring from real strawberries. "Butter and Egg Bread" usually contains yellow dye to make it look as if the bread contains more egg than it really does. Caramel coloring is sometimes added to white bread to make it look like dark, more nutritious whole wheat bread. Such a practice by bakers clearly violates the adulteration law, which forbids the use of additives to make a product "appear better or of greater value than it is," but the FDA has not cracked down.[62] The use of artificial food coloring has increased twenty-fold since 1940 (see Figure 2).[63]

Many artificial colorings are harmful, causing such problems as liver damage and cancer in animal studies. These colorings have been banned. The most recent instance occurred in 1973, when FDA outlawed the coloring called Violet No. 1, which was used in soda pop, candy, and as the "USDA inspected" marking on meat. It was in our food supply for over twenty years—and suspect for at least ten years—before FDA was inspired to act. Violet No. 1 caused cancer in mice, most frequently in females.

Red No. 2, which is now the second most-widely used coloring (more than 900,000 pounds per year in soda pop, candy, gelatin desserts, etc.) is suspected of causing fetal deaths and miscarriages. This suspicion is based on animal studies. For two years FDA has threatened to limit the use of Red No. 2, but has never done so. Anita Johnson, an attorney with Ralph Nader's Health Research Group, has protested vehemently, but the economic interests of the food industry have prevailed over the risks to developing embryos.

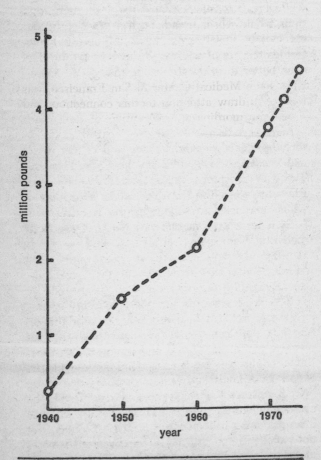

ARTIFICIAL FOOD COLORING PRODUCTION
1940-1974

While cancer and organ damage are among the most dramatic effects, colorings may cause more subtle problems. Several colorings, notably Yellow No. 5, which is the most widely used coloring (1,-289,000 pounds in fiscal year 1974) cause allergic reactions in sensitive people. Colorings (and flavorings) are also suspected of triggering hyperkinetic behavior in children. Dr. Ben Feingold, chief emeritus in the department of allergy at Kaiser-Permanente Medical Center in San Francisco, was the first to draw attention to this connection, and blames the inordinate consumption of junk foods by children for the increasing occurrence of hyperkinesis in school children.[64]

Artificial coloring adds a hazard to food without increasing its nutritional value. Stay away from artificially colored foods. The main exception to this general rule is margarine: the coloring used is carotene, a safe natural product that the body converts to vitamin A.

Sodium nitrite and *sodium nitrate* have been used for centuries in cured meat as colorings, flavorings, and preservatives. They are present in ham, bacon, corned beef, most frankfurters, salami, liverwurst, bologna, and smoked fish. Sodium nitrite can—and sometimes does—combine with other chemicals in meat to form nitrosamines. Extremely tiny amounts of these nitrosamines have caused cancer in animals and almost certainly can cause human cancer. For this reason, nitrite should be avoided. (Nitrate should also be avoided because it breaks down in food to form nitrite.) Fried (but not baked) bacon invariably contains nitrosamines and is the most dangerous nitrite-containing food.[65]

For many foods the meat and fish industries can replace nitrite with other means of preservation, such as sterilization or freezing, but this means added expense and effort, so change is very slow in coming. A few stores sell frozen or refrigerated nitrite-free hot dogs and other sausages, but these products are relatively expensive.

Caffeine occurs naturally in coffee, tea, and chocolate. Cola drinks and Dr. Pepper—as well as many non-prescription drugs—contain added caffeine. Caffeine is a powerful stimulant of the central nervous system—that's why coffee keeps us awake. Too much caffeine, however, will make most people nervous wrecks. Several scientific studies have shown that large amounts of caffeine can cause birth defects in animals. Pregnant women—at least for the first trimester—should avoid caffeine (switch to decaffeinated coffee); the danger is small, but there is no sense in endangering the developing baby unnecessarily.[66]

BHA and *BHT* are synthetic chemicals that are widely used to extend the storage life of oil-containing foods by preventing oils from going rancid. Neither additive is essential. For any food that contains one or both of these additives, a comparable food made by another manufacturer can usually be found without additives. For instance, Wesson oil contains no preservative, while other brands contain several; likewise, Planter's canned peanuts do not have a preservative, while other brands do. If a preservative is deemed necessary, vitamin E is effective and unquestionably safe. BHA and BHT have not been adequately tested, although the tests that have been done do not indicate any hazard—except for occasional allergic reactions.[67]

Cholesterol

Cholesterol is a fat-soluble substance that is the basic building block of sex hormones and other important chemicals in the human body. Cholesterol is present in foods of animal, but never vegetable, origin. It is most abundant in eggs, liver, kidney, and brains (see Table 5). The human liver and intestine produce 500-1000 milligrams of cholesterol a day.

Blood always contains some cholesterol, regardless of how much is present in one's diet. However, studies have shown that the more cholesterol there is in one's diet, the higher the cholesterol level will be in one's blood. Other studies have proven that the risk of coronary heart disease increases greatly as the blood cholesterol level increases. The American Heart Association, American Health Foundation, and many other responsible organizations have urged Americans, particularly young and middle-aged men, to consume no more than an average of 300 milligrams of cholesterol a day (slightly more than is present in one egg).

Eggs and liver are the two most commonly eaten

foods that contain large amounts of cholesterol. They also happen to be two of the most well-balanced and nutritious foods. They are rich in vitamins, high-quality protein, and minerals, and are low in fat. Most women do not have to worry about high cholesterol levels until after menopause and can safely eat eggs and liver. Men, however, show rising cholesterol levels and atherosclerotic blood vessels (the first sign of heart disease) beginning in childhood and adolescence. Boys and men, therefore, should restrict their intake of cholesterol. This does not mean boycotting eggs. A person who is largely vegetarian could safely eat an egg a day. A person who eats meat and drinks several glasses of whole milk in the course of a day could probably eat two or three eggs a week and still meet the Heart Association's 300 milligram guideline. The safest course of action is to visit a doctor or clinic and get your cholesterol level measured. Readers should insist that their friends and relatives do this. Ask your doctor and local chapter of the Heart Association to help you interpret the measurement.

Fish, chicken and beef contain similar levels of cholesterol (see Table 5). Beef, however, contains higher levels of saturated fat than fish or chicken. The high fat content contributes to high cholesterol levels in the consumer's blood. This is why beef is considered a "high cholesterol" food, while chicken and beef are not.

TABLE 5

Cholesterol Content of Common Foods[68]

Food*	Serving Size	Cholesterol (Milligrams)
Milk, skim	1 cup	5
Cottage cheese, uncreamed	½ cup	7
Lard	1 Tbsp.	12
Cream, light table	1 fl. oz.	20
Cottage cheese, creamed	½ cup	24
Cream, half and half	¼ cup	26
Ice cream (approx. 10% fat)	½ cup	27
Cheddar cheese	1 oz.	28
Milk, whole	1 cup	34
Butter	1 Tbsp.	35
Oysters, salmon	3 oz., cooked	40
Clams, halibut, tuna	3 oz., cooked	55
Chicken, light meat	3 oz., cooked	67
Beef, pork, lobster, chicken, dark meat	3 oz., cooked	75
Lamb, veal, crab	3 oz., cooked	85
Shrimp	3 oz., cooked	130
Beef heart	3 oz., cooked	230
Egg	1 yolk or 1 egg	250
Liver, beef, calf, pork, lamb	3 oz., cooked	370
Kidney	3 oz., cooked	680
Brains	3 oz., raw	more than 1700

*Vegetable foods never contain cholesterol.

Organically Grown Food

In the past decade more and more urban Americans have become interested in the way food is grown. Perhaps the proliferation of tasteless, prepared foods—called "plastic" by some—made this phenomenon inevitable. Many people began growing food organically in their gardens or seeking organically grown food in natural food stores. Growing food the organic way means using "natural" fertilizers and "natural" means of controlling insect pests. Organic farmers fertilize their fields with manure and compost, rather than the nitrogen-phosphorus-potassium (NPK) fertilizer that is manufactured in a factory. The preference for the natural is not simply a contempt for factories and a romantic vision of Nature. Compost and manure contain trace elements (which can be, but often aren't, added to NPK fertilizer). Compost also provides humus, which helps hold the soil together. Nitrate-rich fertilizer can be used in excess, with consequent pollution of the local water supply. Most everybody agrees that natural fertilizers are more expensive to use than "chemical" fertilizers, but are significantly healthier for the environment.

Some farmers who rely on insecticides gripe that

they are on a treadmill. They find the more insecticide they use, the greater their insect problem is the following year. Insecticides disrupt the balance of nature, kill the beneficial insects along with the unwanted ones, and may lead to insects that are resistant to pesticides. Many farmers, not just organic farmers, are reducing their reliance on pesticides, using them in minimal quantities and only when needed (as opposed to pre-scheduled, massive sprayings).

Through the years, growers of organic food have devised tricks to prevent insects from devouring their crops. Depending upon the crop, time of year, and region of the country, they have done such things as spray fields with seaweed extract, plant onions or herbs between rows of crops, and import thousands of ladybugs to a field to keep down insect predators. Growing a variety of crops on a small farm, as opposed to raising hundreds of acres of a single crop, maintains a healthy population of predators (birds, insects, spiders, etc.) that helps keep any one pest from disrupting the balance of nature and destroying a crop. Using natural means of controlling pests, instead of malathion, parathion, and the dozens of other synthetic pesticides, keeps our planet cleaner and our food safer.

Organic farming requires more labor and usually results in a smaller yield per acre than standard "chemical farming." Consequently, the price of organically grown food is high. However, in the long run, the higher cost may be a real bargain: as we are finding out, pesticides kill eagles and farm workers in addition to boll weevils; and they add a small hazard to the food we eat. Dieldrin and aldrin, two pesticides that caused cancer in laboratory animals, were banned in 1974, while DDT was banned several years earlier. The challenge to advocates of organic farming is to adapt the small-scale methods to the large farms that supply most of our food. The U.S. Department of Agriculture must assist in this effort, although historically it has been more a hindrance than a help, treating organic farmers as kooks.

Oregon is the first state to recognize the existence of organic farming. The Oregon State Department of Agriculture adopted regulations in 1974 that defined what an "organically grown food" is. Oregon's action may stimulate other states, and eventually the Federal government, to distinguish between organically grown food and other food.

The food rating system used in *Nutrition Scoreboard* does not give any bonus to food grown by organic methods. As yet, there is scanty evidence that this food is more or less nutritious than "agribusiness" food. Only a few limited studies have been conducted and these indicated no nutritional difference between certain vegetables grown organically and by normal methods of farming, but there is inadequate evidence to make any final judgments at this time.

Calories

If people are concerned about any one aspect of foods, surely it is calories. Many nutritionists consider obesity to be America's number one health problem. The surefire path to riches is to write a book on how to lose weight. *The High-Clam, Low-Starch Way to Slimness,* by Dr. X, would be a cinch best-seller. Zillions of calorie counters are sold every year, but oversized bellies seem as prevalent as ever. According to life insurance statistics, between 40 and 70 percent of adults over thirty are 10 percent or more above ideal weight.[3]

The food ratings reflect indirectly the caloric content of food, because our formula penalizes foods that contain more than 20 percent fat or that contain added sugar. We did consider dividing the "nutrient rating" by "calories per serving"—so if two foods had equal amounts of nutrients, the one with fewer calories would have a higher score. However, celery, lettuce, and other foods that have very few calories would have ended up with high "nutrition ratings" even though they contain only tiny amounts of nutrients. We decided that calories and nutrients are both so important that they shouldn't be combined into a single number.

Weight control is far too big and complex a subject to cover in a couple of paragraphs, but is so important that we feel obliged to play Dr. X and dispense a little advice. Dr. Jean Mayer has specialized in the study of obesity and, with his colleagues, has conducted many important studies. One of the most interesting studies showed that workers who have sedentary jobs eat more calories than those whose jobs entail moderate amounts of physical activity.[69] This study highlights the value of exercise to weight control. Not only does exercise use up calories, it also decreases the need for calories (not to mention the fact that jogging, tennis, rowing, gardening, and other activities are fun).

Another study, this conducted by South African scientists, showed that men who ate as little sugar as they could—but made a conscious effort to maintain their weight—lost an average of almost

> "The reduction in energy expenditure because of automation in the United States probably is responsible for part of the increasing incidence of obesity. Of equal importance, however, may be the increasing supply of high calorie food items, and the ability of most persons to purchase these foods . . . The individual willing and able to match caloric intake and output can solve this health problem." Dr. Ogden Johnson, former Director of Nutrition, Food and Drug Administration, 1967.

three pounds over a five-month period. The conclusion from this study is obvious: avoid sugar if you are trying to lose weight.[70]

Finally, remember the roughage! Roughage, or dietary fiber, occurs in whole grain products, fruits, and vegetables. Bran is the richest source of fiber. Dietary fiber binds water as it passes through the digestive system. This causes a full feeling in the stomach and helps control one's appetite. Some dieting aids consist basically of synthetic compounds, like methyl cellulose, that mimic some of the effects of natural fiber. But why buy artificial concoctions, when you can get all the fiber you need from delicious natural foods?

Salt

High intakes of salt, or more specifically the sodium that salt (sodium chloride) contains, is thought by some researchers to cause high blood pressure—hypertension—one of the most serious and widespread health problems. According to Dr. Charles Edwards, then Assistant Secretary for Health (H.E.W.), "hypertension is the primary cause of about sixty thousand deaths a year from stroke and cardiovascular disease."[71] The hypertension-related death rate among blacks is twice that of whites.[72]

According to Dr. Walter Kirkendall, Professor of Medicine at the University of Texas:

The intake of salt among adults in our society varies from 7 to 30 grams or more per day. It is known that nutritional balance for this substance can be achieved with as little as 200 milligrams [0.2 grams] of sodium chloride per day in healthy persons. The discrepancy between need and diet intake of salt is a matter of interest because of the great and unexplained prevalence of hypertension in our society.[73]

For someone who already has high blood pressure, physicians normally prescribe sharply reduced salt intakes. The National Institutes of Health advises that "stringent sodium restricted diets (less than 2 grams per day) bring about some reduction in blood pressure in about one-third of those with hypertension."[74]

All the salt and other sources of sodium (MSG, sodium phosphate, other food additives) in our diet certainly do not contribute to our health and may elevate blood pressure in sensitive individuals. It would be wise—and would not hurt any of us—to reduce our salt intake. Persons whose parents or other close relatives have developed hypertension should make an extra effort to reduce their salt intake. They should also, of course, check their blood pressure periodically.

The Panel on Nutrition and Health of the 1974 Senate hearing on a National Nutrition Policy recommended:

• That persons with hypertension be advised that excess

salt ingestion may make blood pressure elevation worse and that salt restriction may be of great value in treatment.

- That, based on experimental evidence, persons predisposed to hypertension (e.g. those with strong genetic tendencies to high blood pressure) be advised that restriction of salt in diet may be of value in preventing the development of high blood pressure.

The sodium content of some typical foods is listed in Scoreboard 9. Note that natural foods contain very little sodium (at least until we add salt in cooking or at the table), while processed foods contain large amounts. Try to go easy on the salt when you season your food.

SCOREBOARD 9

Sodium Content of Various Foods

Food	Serving Size	Milligrams of Sodium
Nabisco Cream of Wheat, regular	1 oz.	0.5
Wheat flour	1 oz.	1
Orange juice	4 oz.	1
Mazola margarine, unsalted	1 Tbsp.	1
Pear	1	2
Peas	3 oz.	2
Halibut	3 oz.	46
Beef	3 oz.	55

Food	Serving Size	Milligrams of Sodium
Nabisco Cream of Wheat, quick	1 oz.	78.5
Mazola margarine	1 Tbsp.	120
Post Raisin Bran	1 oz.	136
Milk, whole or skim	8 oz.	230
Skippy salted peanuts	¼ cup	310
Pillsbury banana cake	1/12 cake	320
Oscar Mayer bologna	2 oz.	525
Oscar Mayer bacon	3 slices	630
Campbell soups (average)	1 cup	880
Swanson beef 3-course dinner	1	1027
Lipton soups (average)	1 cup	1069
Pillsbury blueberry pancakes	3 (4″) cakes	1125
Swanson meat loaf 3-course dinner	1	2045

Alcohol

Alcoholic beverages are high in calories due to their alcohol and carbohydrate content, but are almost devoid of nutrients. Also, obviously, they are inebriating. Without getting too moralistic, it is clear that alcohol and alcoholism are major problems in the United States:

- Alcohol causes thousands of highway deaths every year
- Nine million American adults display the behavior of alcoholism
- Alcoholism drains the economy of $25 billion a year[75]
- Alcohol, like sugar, squeezes nutrients out of the diet and has no redeeming nutritional value outside of calories[75]
- Heavy drinking greatly increases the risk of cancer of the mouth, larynx, esophagus, and other organs
- Excessive imbibing causes brain and liver damage

Heavy drinkers—persons who consume five or more drinks a day—usually have serious nutritional problems that frequently result in liver or brain damage. According to Dr. Frank Iber, Professor of Medicine at the University of Maryland Medical School, "Fifteen million adults in America consume enough alcohol to account for at least 25% of their daily caloric intake.... The message is that the drinking person needs more nutrients but in fact due to alcohol intake, eats less."[73]

Further, Dr. Iber says that the average alcoholic consumes 10 percent too few calories, one-third too little protein, only half the necessary B-vitamins, and only one-fourth the recommended amount of zinc, magnesium, and phosphorus. To make matters even worse, the alcoholic's poor state of health

TABLE 6

T = trace
... = very small, unmeasurable amounts or none

BEVERAGE	FLUID OUNCES	GRAM WEIGHT	WATER %	ALCOHOL % (BY VOLUME)	FAT (gm)	PROTEIN (gm)	CARBOHYDRATE (gm)	CALCIUM (mg)	IRON (mg)	VITAMIN A (internat. units)	THIAMIN (mg)	RIBOFLAVIN (mg)	NIACIN (mg)	ASCORBIC ACID (mg)	FOOD ENERGY (CALORIES)
BEER	12	360	92	4.5	0	1.0	14	18	T	...	0.01	0.11	2.2	...	150
GIN, RUM, VODKA, OR WHISKEY (86-PROOF)	1.5	42	64	43.0	...	...	T	...	...	...	...	...	...	...	105
DESSERT WINES	3.5	103	77	19.0	0	T	8	8	...	...	0.01	0.02	0.2	...	140
TABLE WINES	3.5	102	86	12.0	0	T	4	9	0.4	...	T	0.01	0.1	...	85
COLA	12	369	90	0.0	0	0.0	37	...	...	0	0.00	0.00	0.0	0	145
FRESH ORANGE JUICE	6	186	88	0.0	.75	1.5	20	20	0.4	375	0.17	0.05	0.8	124	83
TOMATO JUICE	6	186	94	0.0	T	1.5	12	13	1.7	1455	0.09	0.05	1.4	39	50
NONFAT (SKIM) MILK	8	245	87	0.0	T	9.0	12	296	0.1	10	0.09	0.44	0.2	2	90
RECOMMENDED DAILY ALLOWANCES (RDA)						65.0		1000	18.0	5000	1.50	1.70	20.0	60	2800

and need to burn off the alcohol means that his or her nutritional needs are even greater than the average non-drinker's. Alcohol is clearly something that should be consumed in moderation, if at all.

We have not assigned a nutrient value to alcohol, but it would certainly be negative. Table 6 lists the amounts of different nutrients in alcoholic beverages and compares them to the amounts in orange juice, milk, and other beverages.

Foods for Babies

Pregnant women are probably more concerned than any other segment of the population about eating a good diet. They want to ensure that the baby developing within them will enter this world in the best possible health. Unfortunately, the concern for good nutrition before birth is all too often forgotten after birth.

If ordinarily contentious nutritionists can agree upon anything, it is the advisability of breast feeding. Human breast milk is obviously the one food intended specifically for human babies. It is the one food with which humans have evolved over tens of thousands of years. It contains antibodies and enzymes that can reduce the incidence of infections.

It does not cause allergic reactions. It is completely digestible. It contains all the right nutrients needed in the first months of life, and in the proper balance. And it is also inexpensive, convenient, and readily available. Nursing also fills psychological needs of both the mother and baby.

Drs. Samuel Fomon of the University of Iowa and Derrick Jelliffe of UCLA, two eminent pediatric nutritionists, fear that bottle-feeding leads to infant obesity.[76] When babies are fed from a bottle, they say, overfeeding is common, because parents want babies to finish all the milk in the bottle. For breast-fed babies, the meal is over when the baby stops sucking.

Despite the common agreement that breast-feeding is best, fewer than one-fifth of American babies are breast-fed for two months.[77] Too often women leave the hospital planning to breast-feed, only to abandon nursing with a few days or weeks, because of problems that their male doctors do not know how to solve. Modern medicine's attitude toward breast-feeding has been, "if for any reason it doesn't work, switch immediately to the bottle." This is a very unscientific approach. There are few difficulties that cannot be quickly alleviated. After all, in the less developed nations, virtually all mothers successfully nurse their babies. Mothers in the U.S. receive little active encouragement to nurse their babies. Nurses at hospitals do not want to be bothered bringing the baby to the mother . . . it is much more expedient to feed the baby from a bottle every few hours. Doctors know little about the merits of breast-feeding, because medical schools barely even treat this subject. Also, doctors, most of whom are male, are often shy about discussing breast-feeding. Lovely full-page ads in magazines intended for new mothers tout the merits of canned formula, comparing it favorably with breast milk. Of course, there are no comparable commercial interests to run ads for breast-feeding. New mothers are generally given a free six-pack of canned formula when they leave the hospital. Finally, government-funded health clinics and hospitals frequently distribute literature donated by the makers of canned formula. The literature contains ads for and all kinds of advice about canned formula; lip service is sometimes given to the merits of breast-feeding, but the name of the game is selling formula.

In the last few years, there has been a trend back to breast-feeding, primarily among college-educated women. They are recognizing that the age-old practice of breast-feeding offers psychological and physiological benefits that bottle-feeding cannot match. Women who are thinking of breast-feeding their babies should contact the local chapter or national office of La Leche League International (9616 Minneapolis Ave., Franklin Park, Illinois 60131) for sensible information and moral support ("leche" is the Spanish word for milk). The League is particularly helpful when a woman has trouble nursing.

Most babies are ready for and need solid foods after about four to six months of nursing. Most mothers start their children on solid foods much earlier, often to demonstrate to grandparents and friends that their children are progressing rapidly. There is, however, no good purpose in feeding a

119

baby solid food too early. Solid food is less nutritious than milk, and some varieties are higher in calories. Most doctors, not knowing much about nutrition, do not discourage the premature use of solid foods. When your baby is ready for solid foods, you can either mash and strain your own or buy the more expensive commercially prepared foods. After a few months of this food, your baby's teeth will have started coming in, and you can switch to mashed-up, ordinary table food.

Most commercial baby foods are made by taking ordinary foods, mashing them up, diluting them with water, adding sugar and salt (these seasonings may lead to overeating and obesity), then frequently adding starch to form a thick slurry. The starch masks the presence of all the added water and is, according to the author's interpretation of the Federal Food, Drug and Cosmetic Act, an adulterant. The starch's empty calories replace fruit, meat, vegetables, and other more valuable ingredients.

If you buy commerically prepared foods, you will notice that junk foods are as much a part of the baby food industry as of other segments of the food industry. In an attempt to gain additional shelf space, companies have come out with all kinds of sugary desserts (e.g. Gerber's raspberry cobbler and Heinz's apple pie). These products have little redeeming nutritional merit and should not be fed to babies. Complain as they may, nutritionists inside and outside of the companies have little influence compared to the marketing specialists. The FDA has not made any attempts to issue regulations that would prevent the proliferation of products that are not healthful to the tiny consumers. By making your own baby foods, you can avoid the sugar and starch that are present in most commercial baby foods. One good book on the subject is *Making Your Own Baby Foods*, by James and Mary Turner (Bantam Books, New York, 1973).

The three major baby food manufacturers, Gerber, Heinz, and Beech-Nut, have all refused to disclose how much sugar and starch they add to their foods. For this reason, we have not been able to calculate nutritional scores. In general, judging from the labels, Gerber's foods seem to be slightly more nutritious than Heinz's or Beech-Nut's. Avoid the sugary foods. And do not feed your baby solid foods too early.

You can feed your baby regular table foods after its teeth develop. Do not waste your money on the commercial "junior foods" or "toddler meals."

IV. Limitations of the Rating System

LIKE ANY SIMPLE system, our food rating system is not perfect. The major flaw is that the rating does not indicate which nutrients contribute how many points. Thus, two foods with similar ratings could be entirely dissimilar. Milk (39) and tomato juice (37), for instance, have similar ratings, but totally different nutrient contents. Milk contains generous amounts of protein, calcium, riboflavin, and vitamin A, while tomato juice contains large amounts of vitamins A and C and small amounts of several other nutrients. You could drink tomato juice until you turned blue in the face, but you would die of malnutrition unless you obtained protein, calcium, and riboflavin from milk or other foods.

Another shortcoming of the rating system is that while it gives equal weight to each of nine nutrients, some of the nutrients are worth more to certain people. Thus, a low income Spanish-American in the southern United States may consume too little vitamin C while a black neighbor may consume too little thiamin. These persons would obviously not be helped by drinking a quart of milk a day, which despite its high score contains little of the needed nutrients. The special needs of a single individual are not easily incorporated into a simple formula and so we gave equal weight to each of five vitamins, two minerals, and protein. As Professor Harris wrote in his paper on the comparative values of different breads, "Since all nutrients are equally essential in the nutrition of human beings, each was given equal importance in calculating the relative over-all nutritional ratings."[14]

A few people may think that to have a nutritious, balanced diet all they have to do is consume the appropriate amounts of certain vitamins, minerals, and protein every day. They may pop a vitamin-mineral supplement or gulp down an Instant Breakfast to start the day and devour a large steak to satisfy their protein requirement at the end of the day. In between they might consume six bottles of soda pop, four candy bars, several cups of coffee, a six-pack of beer, seven doughnuts, and a couple of Hunt's Snack-Pack imitation puddings. Obviously, this diet will look good if you just look at the intake of vitamins, minerals, and protein. Equally obviously, this is a rotten diet. A slug of vitamins and minerals will not automatically counterbalance the detrimental effects of enormous amounts of sugar, alcohol, and fat any more than painting the outside of a house and using a lawnmower will correct an ugly interior. Our goal should be a diet composed of good foods, foods that will provide us with generous amounts of all the necessary nutrients—not just the cheap ones that are sprayed on breakfast cereals or included in pills. The makings of a good diet can be obtained from most grocery stores: fruits, vegetables, dairy products, beans, nuts, whole wheat bread and brown rice, meat, poultry, and fish. If the store

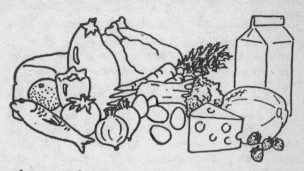

where you shop does not carry such basic foods as whole wheat bread and brown rice, complain to the manger and patronize a store that does. Having an occasional soft drink or candy bar is not harmful, but it's easy to get hooked on the sugary snacks that the junk food pushers tempt us with. A diet comprised of good foods provides our bodies with generous amounts of most nutrients, supplies the fiber and trace minerals that are rarely present in pills, will contain any undiscovered nutrients, should contain few chemical additives, and probably will TASTE GREAT.

A final problem to point out is that manufacturers are increasingly adding nutrients to fabricated foods, and these nutrients are usually precisely the ones that are included in the rating system. They were selected for use in our formula because they are often the only ones that are reported in analyses of foods. Fortification may result in high scores for foods that are clearly undesirable because of their high caloric content and lack of trace minerals, protein, and fiber. As Dr. Jean Mayer has said:

But, unfortunately, many people are getting a false sense of security from food enrichment. And many nutritionists, like me, are worried about it. Enrichment is fine as far as it goes, but by itself it doesn't guarantee a healthy diet. Quite a few necessary vitamins and minerals are excluded from any enrichment program.[78]

Until fortification became widespread, the vitamins and minerals that are used in this rating system were fairly good indicators of overall nutritional worth. If one or more of these nutrients was present in a reasonable quantity, it was likely that significant amounts of other nutrients, such as magnesium, vitamin B-6, potassium, and fiber, were also present. That is no longer the case since companies began manufacturing foods from purified chemicals; they add a limited number of nutrients to a food based on oil, sugar, water, and additives. Fortification can sometimes fool the formula, but you can stay ahead of the game by shunning vitamin-coated junk foods, like Hostess Twinkies, Count Chocula, Kaboom, and Breakfast Squares, all of which contain gobs of sugar. Try to base your diet on basic, untampered-with foods.

I believe that the overall validity of the rating system far outweighs the limitations just described. Developing the rating system has improved my eating habits. I sincerely hope that reading these pages will do the same for yours.

V. The Nutritional Ratings of Common Foods

THE SCOREBOARDS ON the following pages list the relative nutritional values of many common foods. In general, the higher the rating the more nutritious the food. Eat more of the foods near the tops of the charts; eat less of the foods that have negative ratings or are near the bottoms of the charts. Small differences in ratings (for example, 34 versus 36) are not really significant.

The ratings give positive credit to protein, unsaturated fat, starch and naturally occurring sugars, five vitamins, two minerals, trace elements, and fiber (roughage). A food loses points for saturated fat, a fat content above 36 percent of the calories, and added sugar and corn syrup.

All ratings were calculated for one "average" serving of food. In most cases the scores of larger or smaller servings are simply proportional to the standard rating. Thus, while one plum has a score of 9, two plums receive 18 points. Three cups of coffee with sugar have a score of −36, triple the rating of one cup. Half a box of Cracker Jack has a score of −20, one-half the score of a whole box. There are exceptions to this rule, though, because no food is given more than 50 points per nutrient. Thus, a 4-ounce glass of orange juice receives 50 points for its vitamin C; an 8-ounce serving contains twice as much vitamin C, theoretically worth 100 points. But the maximum allowed for a single vitamin is 50 points. Thus, the score for 8 ounces of O. J. is not 124 (2 times 62), but only 74. (50 plus 2 times 12). The score for a food like milk, on the other hand, does double when the serving doubles, because the 39 points for 8 ounces are contributed by moderate amounts of many nutrients.

Important Notice: Eat a Variety of Foods

Stick to the top foods in the various categories. In the beverages, for instance, don't drink just milk, because this and all other foods lack important nutrients—no food is perfect. Among other nutrients, milk lacks iron, fiber, and vitamin C. Drink variety. Restricting your diet to one or two basic foods—brown rice for macrobiotics, tuna or swordfish for weight-watchers—increases greatly the risks of malnutrition and poisoning. A New York woman was on a reducing diet and ate swordfish, swordfish, and more swordfish. After a while this previously healthy woman began to experience dizziness, lapses of memory, difficulty in focusing

> "There's a whole generation of Americans that doesn't know what food tastes like. Their concept of normality is a Hostess Twinkie." Nancy Polatty, 1973.

her eyes, and other problems. Doctors determined that she was being poisoned by the small amounts of mercury in the fish. The mercury was not enough to harm the average eater, but she consumed ten ounces of swordfish a day over a long period of time. Eat variety. Liver and spinach are both fine foods and contain lots of vitamin A. But if you ate just spinach, liver, and carrots every day, you might suffer the headaches and fatigue that are symptomatic of vitamin A poisoning. Vitamin A is great, but too much of a great thing is not always great. Eat variety. But limit that variety to good foods.

Brand names are included for illustrative purposes. In general, the most widely distributed, well-known products were selected. That a food was or was not named is in no way intended to imply an endorsement or criticism.

The ratings of different foods can be added. For instance, a hamburger sandwich would have a rating of 54 (hamburger = 34; bun = 18; catsup = 2). If a food is not listed, use the rating for a similar food. While the ratings of foods can be added, there is no magic goal to shoot for. A diet adding up to 750 or 1,000 points a day is almost certainly balanced, but it still might lack certain nutrients.

One unavoidable problem with any book that mentions brand names is that new products are always being added, products that do not sell are dropped, and others are modified. Many products aimed at children are dropped as children tire of them or of the TV shows on which they are advertised. In the past two years General Mills has stopped making Sir Grapefellow and Baron Von

Redberry cereals, General Foods has dumped Pink Panther Flakes, and Hunt-Wesson has dropped "snack pack" gelatin desserts. Candy companies routinely adjust the sizes of their candy bars, as raw material and labor costs vary . . . and in the past few years candy bars have shrunk in size and risen in price. Another trend is for manufacturers to fortify their products with vitamins and minerals to neutralize the criticism of nutritionists (if not the effects of a high sugar content). Because of these periodic product changes, the scores of a few foods may have changed between the time the scores were calculated and the time you read this book.

Soups

Soup is a good way of getting the old taste buds geared up for one of the thousand-odd meals we eat every year. Usually we select soup on the basis of flavor and variety, but as Scoreboard 13 shows, it is an easy matter to make nutrition one of the criteria we use to select a soup.

We have rated only one homemade soup (see recipe), because recipes vary widely. Homemade soups can be extremely nutritious and delicious, and an economical way of using left overs. At the Center for Science in the Public Interest, we take turns making thick and (usually) delicious soups several times a week. It takes only a few minutes to prepare ingredients and dump them into a big pot of boiling, salted water ... and then let the

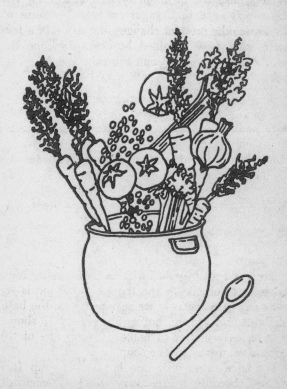

Lentil-Tomato Soup

1 pound dried lentils
    (about 2¼ cups)
8 cups water   Optional Seasonings:
1 large onion, chopped
6 carrots, chopped   2 bay leaves
3 celery stalks, chopped   1 tsp. sweet basil
1 large can tomatoes   1 tsp. thyme
    (1 lb., 12 oz. can)
1½ tsp. salt
½ tsp. pepper

Put all ingredients and spices, except the tomatoes, into a large pot and simmer for 3 hours. Add more water if the soup gets too thick. Stir in the tomatoes at the end. Makes 11 cups.

soup simmer for about two hours. Ingredients may include carrots, a soup bone, brown rice, lentils, beans, cabbage, chicken, split peas, and mushrooms. Adding fresh or canned tomatoes will make almost any soup taste good. Experiment with just about any food in your refrigerator or cupboards. Making soup can be an exciting after-school adventure for children—and a way of getting them interested in cooking and eating nourishing foods.

In the past couple of years, the major soupmakers have opened up a new market by producing soups that contain large amounts of meat and vegetables. Some of these soups are so thick that many people probably eat them instead of part or all of a main course. The Campbell Chunky soups and a couple of the Heinz Great American soups are quite nutritious. The major reason for the high ratings of Chunky Turkey, Chunky Vegetable, Chunky Beef, and Great American Vegetarian Vegetable soups is that they have between 90 and 100 percent of the RDA for vitamin A—this derived mainly from carrots. In addition, the Chunky meat soups and Great American Hearty Vegetable Beef soup receive between 8 and 12 points for protein—this represents between 16 and 24 percent of a person's RDA for protein—quite a bit for a canned soup.

Clearly the least nutritious soups are the good old-fashioned bouillon, consommé, chicken noodle, chicken with rice, and onion soups. These have little protein (chicken noodle soup can contain as little as 2 percent chicken!) and only small amounts of the various vitamins and minerals. Tomato, vegetable beef, vegetarian vegetable, and chili beef—not to mention good homemade soups—are far better buys as far as nutrition goes.

New England clam chowder is made with half a can of milk and the score includes the milk. All the other condensed soups are prepared with water.

SCOREBOARD 10
Canned Soups
(One cup serving)

	NUTRITIONAL SCORE
Lentil-tomato (homemade)	99
Campbell Chunky Turkey	76

	NUTRITIONAL SCORE
Campbell Chunky Vegetable	69
Heinz Great American Vegetarian Vegetable	68
Campbell Chunky Beef	63
Heinz Great American Vegetable Beef	46
Campbell vegetable beef	45
Campbell tomato	42
Campbell turkey vegetable	42
Campbell Chunky Chicken	39
Campbell vegetarian vegetable	39
Heinz Great American Split Pea and Smoked Ham*	36
Campbell New England clam chowder	34
Campbell chili beef	34
Lipton vegetable beef	24
Campbell Manhattan style clam chowder	22
Heinz Great American Chicken Noodle and Dumplings	16
Campbell turkey noodle	15
Campbell Chicken with Stars	15
Lipton turkey noodle	12
Campbell chicken noodle	10
Campbell chicken with rice	9
Lipton chicken noodle "cup-a-soup"	9
Campbell onion soup	8
Campbell beef broth (bouillon)	8
Campbell consommé	8

*This food contains sodium nitrite, an additive that should be avoided.

Non-Dairy Beverages

The difference between a well-balanced meal and a deficient one often lies in the drink that washes it down. Three of the best drinks are milk (rich in protein, calcium, and riboflavin), orange juice (rich in vitamin C, small amounts of vitamin A and B-vitamins), and tomato juice (generous amounts of vitamins A and C). These drinks can make a major contribution to the nutritional value of a meal.

Of course, not everyone drinks the Big Three. Soft drinks and coffee, which are dispensed by zillions of vending machines and promoted by enormous advertising expenditures, are often drunk in place of nutritious alternatives. In 1972 the average American drank 36 gallons of coffee, 30 gallons of soda pop, 25 gallons of milk, and 20 gallons of beer.[79]

Coffee and tea contain no nutrients, but do contain caffeine which, being a powerful stimulant of the central nervous system, can keep you awake and make you jittery if you are sensitive or drink too much. The score for coffee and tea is knocked from 0 to −12 by the addition of a teaspoon of sugar. Keeping a good supply of cold water, good

135

soup, and fruit juices at home and in the office can help you break that coffee habit.

Worse than coffee are the soft drinks. These contain only sugar, water, acid, artificial coloring, and a few other goodies—none of which is nutritious. In addition, cola drinks and Dr. Pepper contain caffeine, which has the same drug-like effect on our nervous system as the caffeine in coffee. But the worst aspect of soft drinks is the sugar content, and it is that that drives the score down to −92 for a 12-ounce serving. The per capita consumption of soft drinks in the United States has doubled in the past eleven years (see Figure 3). A survey taken several years ago by *Boys Life* magazine revealed that their average Boy Scout reader consumed more than three 8-ounce servings of soda pop a day (in August). Eight percent of the boys drank eight or more servings a day! This much soda pop supplies between one-third and one-fourth of a boy's daily

"A recently controlled experiment with children who consumed 12 ounces of soft drink a day for 3 years showed that they suffered in certain teeth 50-150 percent more decay than another group who drank water. On the whole, the decay rate tended to be higher in the soft drink consuming group compared with the water-drinking group." Dr. Abraham Nizel, School of Dental Medicine, Tufts University, 1973.

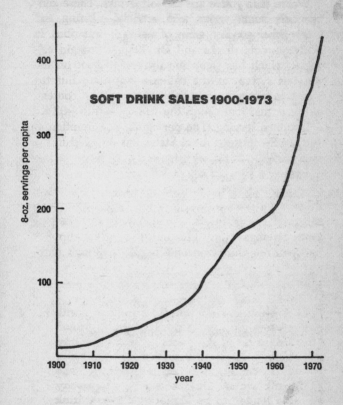

SOFT DRINK SALES 1900-1973

8-oz. servings per capita

400

300

200

100

1900 1910 1920 1930 1940 1950 1960 1970

year

caloric requirement—and squeezes a good fraction of nutritious foods out of the diet. Kool-Aid contains a great amount of sugar, and even though it is fortified with vitamin C it still has a wretched score of −55 for an 8-ounce serving.

Artificially-sweetened soft drinks contain saccharin instead of sugar and provide almost no calories. The absence of sugar is great, but the safety of saccharin is questionable. The FDA is currently reviewing animal studies in which large amounts of saccharin caused tumors. If you want a cheap, refreshing, low-calorie drink, why not reach for a glass of tomato juice (50 calories per 6 ounces) or good old-fashioned water?

Chemists are busily working away in their labs devising factory-made substitutes for orange juice. General Foods' attempts in this field, Orange Plus, Awake, and Tang, have significantly lower scores than the real thing. Tang and orange juice have

"The per capita consumption of soft drinks must be in the neighborhood of more than three (6-oz.) bottles a week . . . It seems obvious that, regardless of the method used to estimate the amount of sugar consumed as soft drinks, one obtains a result that is definitely undesirable from the standpoint of the nation's nutritional welfare." (1973 consumption of soft drinks is triple what it was in 1942.) Council on Foods and Nutrition, American Medical Association, 1942.

equal amounts of vitamin C; Orange Plus and Awake have only one-third as much vitamin C as O.J.; and all three ersatz drinks are totally devoid of riboflavin and niacin, of which O.J. has small amounts. In addition, Tang loses 37 points, Awake loses 31 points, and Orange Plus loses 19 points because of the added sugar. Finally, the imitation orange drinks contain artificial coloring, which we should avoid whenever possible.

SCOREBOARD 11
Non-Dairy Beverages

FOOD	SERVING SIZE	NUTRITIONAL SCORE
Orange juice	4 oz.	62
V-8 juice	4 oz.	40
Tomato juice	4 oz.	37
Tang (fortified)	4 oz.	30
Orange Plus (fortified)	4 oz.	20
Awake (fortified)	4 oz.	10
Apple juice	4 oz.	7
Hi-C (fortified)	4 oz.	3
Coffee with cream*	8 oz.	1
Coffee or tea*	8 oz.	0
Artificially sweetened soda pop	12 oz.	0
Coffee with sugar*	8 oz.	− 9
Kool-Aid (fortified)	8 oz.	−55
Soda pop*	12 oz.	−92

*Coffee, tea, and cola beverages contain caffeine.

Dairy Products

As the National Dairy Council is fond of telling us, dairy products are among the most nutritious and well-rounded foods available—for most people. Milk is one of the best sources of calcium, riboflavin, and protein. An 8-ounce glass contains about 19 percent of our daily allotment of protein, 29 percent of the calcium we need, and 24 percent of the riboflavin. Milk also contains some vitamin A and thiamin.

The main problem with milk is that it contains saturated fat, which appears to contribute to the development of heart disease. Your best bet is to get your blood cholesterol level measured to see whether or not you have a problem. Until you visit a doctor, or if you have a high level, you can play it safe by buying low-fat milk (1 or 2 percent butterfat), skim milk (0 percent), or buttermilk (0 percent); whole milk has 3.5-4 percent fat. Women who have reached menopause and men, in particular, should be concerned about fat and cholesterol.

A second problem relates to lactose, the main carbohydrate in milk. In most white Americans and Europeans, an enzyme in the small intestine breaks lactose into its two component sugars, glucose and galactose, which are then absorbed into the bloodstream and used for energy. Research in recent years has shown that most people, especially blacks and orientals, lose that enzyme during childhood and are not able to digest the lactose. Instead, bacteria in the large intestine metabolize the lactose. This causes flatulence (intestinal gas), diarrhea, and stomachaches. It may, at first, seem unusual to white Americans that a large percentage of humans cannot drink milk comfortably, but, in fact, few adult mammals drink milk (the domestic cat is one obvious exception). Before lactose intolerance was recognized, powdered milk was a staple in America's foreign aid program. Latin American, African, and Asian recipients who could not drink milk used the free powder for whitewashing houses, as a laxative, or simply threw it away.

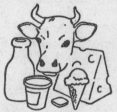

Yogurt is made by adding certain bacteria to milk, usually low-fat milk. As the bacteria multiply they convert some of the lactose (milk sugar) to lactic acid. The acid curdles the milk and adds flavor. Yogurt has all the nutrition of the milk, but can be stored for a much longer time. The score of 44 is for plain low-fat yogurt. Adding sugar or preserves, as is often done commercially or by the consumer, lowers the score considerably. If you've never had yogurt, try a cup—you're in for a pleasant, refreshing surprise.

Cottage cheese (creamed or uncreamed) is one of the best foods around. A half-cup serving contains about one-third of our daily protein requirement and 17 percent of our riboflavin requirement. Mix cottage cheese with raisins, diced peaches, or pineapple if you want a touch of sweetness. Most other cheeses are not quite as good as cottage cheese, because of their high content of saturated fat: cheddar loses 14 points, and American loses 18 points. However, they still have good scores because they are rich sources of protein, riboflavin, calcium, and vitamin A. A 2-ounce serving of Swiss cheese, for instance, contains 30 percent of the daily dose of protein, half of the calcium requirement, and 13 percent each of the vitamin A and riboflavin allotments—not bad for two ounces of food.

The least nutritious of the cheeses listed is cream cheese. Its score of zero is due to a balancing out between small amounts of protein and vitamin A on the one hand and a high fat content on the other. A cottage cheese and lox sandwich would be much more nutritious than cream cheese and lox, but I am not sure how good it would taste.

Ice cream is the least nutritious of the milk-derived products. A 3-ounce serving contains relatively little calcium (7 percent of the RDA), vitamins, and protein. On the other hand it contains saturated fat (-3) and a lot of sugar (-25). Ice cream is fine to eat on special occasions, but not so good if you eat it (and other high-sugar, high-fat foods) too frequently.

Cream has a score of 1. A tablespoon has a bit of protein, vitamin A, and calcium (1 point each). But this is balanced by a high fat content. Despite cream's fat content, it is still a better nutritional buy than imitation coffee whitener (containing coconut oil which is a saturated fat), which has a score of −5. The reason for the difference is that the imitation product has no vitamins or minerals, and has a little sugar (−2.5 points). Cream and coffee whitener both lose 3 points for saturated fat. Coffee whiteners made with polyunsaturated oil are just coming on the market.

SCOREBOARD 12

Dairy Products

Food	Serving Size	Nutritional Score
Skim milk	8 oz.	49
Buttermilk	8 oz.	45
Yogurt, lowfat (no preserves)	8 oz.	44
Swiss cheese	2 oz.	43
Whole milk	8 oz.	39
Cheddar cheese	2 oz.	38
Cottage cheese, creamed	½ cup	34
Cottage cheese, uncreamed	½ cup	32
American cheese	2 oz.	32
Cream	¾ oz.	1
Cream cheese	½ oz.	0

Food	Serving Size	Nutritional Score
Butter	1 pat	− 3
Coffee whitener (made with coconut oil)	¾ oz.	− 5
Ice cream	3 oz.	−18

Vegetables

What is it about vegetables that causes so many children to turn up their noses? Spinach, ugh. Asparagus, ugh. Potato, ugh. Fortunately, in adulthood most people realize that a well-cooked vegetable is truly a gift from the gods. The tender tips of asparagus ... the succulent leaves of artichoke protecting the ineffably delicious heart ... the crisp crunch of the carrot ... the fragrant and delicate buds on broccoli looking like tiny leaves on a miniature tree ... the tomato, that red treasure, picked at the peak of lusciousness from the backyard garden.

Vegetables come in as many sizes, shapes, flavors, and textures as one could ever want. And what's more, most vegetables are highly nutritious. Collard and turnip greens, kale, broccoli, and spinach head the list, each with a score over 100. There is only one word for these vegetables: incredible. A single serving of each of these supplies 100 percent of our daily need for vitamin A (50 points). In addition, broccoli spears, kale, and collard greens supply 100 percent of the recommended allotment of vitamin C (50 points); spinach and turnip greens supply upwards of 60 percent of our daily need for vitamin C. These four vegetables also contain moderate amounts of the B-vitamins. Collard and turnip greens, kale, and spinach receive between 5 and 8 points for their calcium content. However, spinach leaves contain oxalic acid which combines with some of the calcium and prevents it from being absorbed.

A colorful sweet potato (87) is more nutritious than its albino cousins, the baked (33) and boiled (26) potato. All three contain about 33 percent of the RDA of vitamin C (it was this vitamin C that prevented the Irish and other Northern peoples from developing scurvy). In addition, a serving of sweet potato supplies 100 percent of the body's daily need for vitamin A, for which it receives 50 points. Keep a few boiled potatoes in your refrigerator at all times; they make excellent snacks and can be eaten for breakfast, lunch, or dinner. Romaine lettuce, which has a deep green color, outshines iceberg lettuce. Romaine has three times as much calcium, iron, and vitamin C and six times as much vitamin A as iceberg. The score of romaine is 28, iceberg 10.

Cook vegetables in a minimum of water to preserve their food value and flavor, cook only until tender crisp, and serve them attractively.

Spinach, chard, fresh corn on the cob, broccoli, cauliflower, and mushrooms can all be eaten raw.

The least nutritious—but still wholesome and nutritious—of the commonly eaten vegetables is corn. Despite its relatively poor showing (a serving contains between 5 and 10 percent of the RDA of vitamin C and several B vitamins), Americans love corn and so it is widely used in frozen dinners. Peas, although no match for spinach or broccoli, would be a far more nutritious ingredient than corn. A serving of peas contains between 10 and 23 percent of the RDA of vitamins A and C, thiamin, riboflavin, and niacin—quite a nice balance.

Holding down the bottom of the chart are beets, celery, lettuce, and cucumber. They contain fiber and a small amount of other nutrients, mainly vitamin C. They are fine if you like their taste, but other vegetables are more nutritious.

One of the shortcomings of McDonald's and most other fast-food chains is that the only vegetable they serve is potato. Meals are woefully deficient in vitamin A. McDonald's has advertised that a meal of a milk shake, order of fries, and two hamburgers supplies only 6 percent of one's daily vitamin A requirement. Burger Chef recently began installing salad bars in their shops, an innovation that deserves applause. You can pile as much lettuce and tomato on your hamburger or tray as you want. Don't be shy about going back for seconds or thirds. Hopefully, other chains will follow Burger Chef's example.

By sticking to vegetables closer to the top of the chart than the bottom, you should be able to increase greatly your intake of vitamins A and C.

Eat broccoli, spinach, collard and turnip greens, kale, brussel sprouts, and peas. Serve sweet potato in place of white potato occasionally. Eat a tomato (which contains generous amounts of vitamin A and C) as a snack or add it to some of your dishes. If the tomatoes are hard, fleshy, and tasteless where you shop, try canned tomatoes or grow your own. Buy whole, instead of chopped, spinach and broccoli. Buy frozen vegetables without the yukky cream sauce; the sauce is expensive and sometimes replaces the vegetable. The main thing, though, is to eat a lot of vegetables, of any kind. They are all fine foods.

Children who turn up their noses at the mere mention of vegetables are missing out on real treats. The best way of interesting your children in vegetables is to encourage them to make a small garden in the backyard. Children are thrilled as they follow the miraculous development of a tiny seed into a mature plant. And few children will not eat the tomato, peas, or swiss chard that they

"The diet consumed in the United States —high in animal products and in highly processed foods—may be not only expensive and inefficient to produce but nutritionally unsound. If so, our current problems in educating people and modifying dietary practices will seem modest compared with those in the future." Prof. D. Mark Hegsted, Dept. of Nutrition, Harvard School of Public Health.

"Rice & Vegetable Nirvana"

. . . A fantastic main course . . . this recipe makes 4 servings

A) The Rice. Prepare 4 cups of brown rice, (1⅜ cups rice, 2⅝ cups water). Add ⅓ cup of raisins a few minutes before removing from heat. Add curry or other spice if you desire.

B) The Vegies. Get a large frying pan (several inches deep) and a cutting board. Cut up the following and cook gently (cover the pan) in a bit of oil and the vegetables' juices:

> 6 medium sized carrots (cut into discs or strips)
> 2 green peppers
> 1 pound of fresh broccoli
> 3 tomatoes (cut in sixths or eighths)
> ½ cup shelled, unsalted peanuts

Don't be limited by this recipe; add celery, bean sprouts, cauliflower, apple, or what have you. Season with salt, pepper, and other spices.

C) Serving. Serve the vegies on a bed of rice. For your beverage try orange, tomato, or V-8 juice or milk. Also, be sure to have heated up a fresh loaf of whole-wheat bread.

For dessert have cantaloupe or watermelon. Brace yourself for an incredibly delicious, nutrition-packed meal.

themselves grew. Also, no vegetable tastes better than a home-grown one. In some cities schools use a local park or arboretum to introduce students to the pleasures of growing vegetables. If you cannot work out a garden arrangement, have your children help prepare and cook fresh vegetables.

SCOREBOARD 13
Vegetables

FOOD	SERVING SIZE*	NUTRITIONAL SCORE
Collard greens**	3⅓ oz.	126
Kale, with stems and midribs	3⅓ oz.	118
Broccoli**	3⅓ oz.	116
Turnip greens	3⅓ oz.	111
Spinach**	3⅓ oz.	104
Spinach, chopped**	3⅓ oz.	91
Broccoli, chopped**	3⅓ oz.	83
Sweet potato, baked	3⅓ oz.	82
Peas and carrots**	3⅓ oz.	80
Mixed vegetables**	3⅓ oz.	77
Brussels sprouts**	3⅓ oz.	73
Tomato, raw	1	69
Spinach, creamed**	3⅓ oz.	68
Carrots, canned	3⅓ oz.	59
Cauliflower**	3⅓ oz.	54
Peas**	3⅓ oz.	52
Asparagus	3⅓ oz.	49
Cabbage, chopped	1 cup	48
Lima beans, baby**	3⅓ oz.	41

Food	Serving Size*	Nutritional Score
Avocado, summer (Fla.)	½	40
Peas, canned	3⅓ oz.	36
Potatoes, french fried	2½ oz.	34
Potato, baked, no skin	3⅓ oz.	32
Lettuce, romaine	2 oz.	28
Artichoke	½ bud	27
Green pepper	¼ pod	25
Potato, boiled without peel	3⅓ oz.	25
Green beans, cut**	3⅓ oz.	25
Sauerkraut, canned	½ cup	25
Turnips, diced	½ cup	23
Corn, kernel**	3⅓ oz.	23
Zucchini squash, boiled	3⅓ oz.	22
Avocado, winter (Calif.)	½	21
Green beans, canned	3⅓ oz.	23
Potato, mashed, with butter	3⅓ oz.	20
Okra	4 pods	19
Corn, kernel, canned	3⅓ oz.	18
Beets, diced	3⅓ oz.	13
Radishes	4	12
Lettuce, iceberg	2 oz.	10
Cucumber	six ⅛″ slices	8
Celery	8″ x 1½″	7
Onion	¼ of a 2½″	6

*3⅓ oz. and ½ cup are approximately equal.
**Frozen.

Fresh Fruits

All fruits are good and nutritious. They make great snacks and fine desserts. Keep several kinds of fruit on hand at all times—and treat your friends to a colorful surprise when they visit you.

As Scoreboard 14 shows, different fruits have very different nutritional values. Up at the top of the chart is cantaloupe, an amazingly nutritious fruit. One-fourth of an average-sized melon receives 49 points for vitamin A (98 percent of the RDA) and 39 points for vitamin C (78 percent of the RDA). The runner-up spot goes to watermelon—and this is a surprise to most people, even nutritionists. Almost everyone thinks that watermelon is not nutritious, perhaps because children like it so much. How wrong they are. An average-sized wedge (two pounds including the heavy rind) supplies half of the recommended intake of both vitamins A and C (25 points each), has a fair amount of carbohydrate (6 points, the same as a banana), and contains more iron per serving than any other fruit on the chart (3 points). Eat watermelon both for good taste and good nutrition.

The high scores for strawberries, grapefruit, tan-

gerine, and pineapple are due largely to their high
vitamin C content. A peach, on the other hand, has
twice as much vitamin A as C (13 points versus 6
points).

An apple a day keeps the doctor away, and all
that, but still it contains just a small amount of vitamins (5 percent of the RDA for vitamin C, for
example) and a moderate amount of carbohydrate
(5 points). Its score is only 12. However, a good
apple is crisp and crunchy, contains valuable fiber,
and helps clean the teeth. The pectin and other fiber in the apple helps reduce blood cholesterol
levels. Keep a bag of apples in the refrigerator for
snacks and for guests.

SCOREBOARD 14

Fresh Fruits

FOOD	SERVING SIZE	NUTRITIONAL SCORE
Cantaloupe	¼ melon	99
Watermelon	2 lbs.*	74
Orange	1	68
Honeydew melon	¼ melon	59
Strawberries	½ cup	50
Grapefruit	½	45
Pineapple, diced	1 cup	35
Tangerine	1	34
Peach	1	29
Banana	1	26
Pear	1	20

Food	Serving Size	Nutritional Score
Apricot	1	18
Blueberries	½ cup	16
Prunes	4	16
Cherries	10	15
Apple	1	12
Grapes	1 cup	12
Plum	1	9

*This weight includes the rind; however, any nutrients in the rind were not included in the score.

Protein Foods

The body needs protein daily to replace dead cells and to build new cells, enzymes, and hair. Muscle cells are made largely of protein. The body makes the proteins it needs from the protein in food. Poultry, fish, and red meat are rich in high quality protein, as are dairy products and soybeans.

Aside from providing protein, many foods listed in Scoreboard 15 are good sources of iron. Iron is an important component of hemoglobin, the molecule in red blood cells that carries oxygen to all parts of the body. Blood and meat are red because of the iron that they contain. Meat, dried beans and most of the other foods in this Scoreboard (except for peanut butter, eggs, and bacon) contain a considerable amount of iron, one of the hardest-to-get nutrients. Iron deficiency is partly responsible for the high incidence of anemia in the United States.

As the Scoreboard shows, nutritional values of protein sources vary tremendously. The scores range from a lofty 172 for a 2-ounce serving of beef liver to a lowly 2 for a 2-ounce serving of bologna.

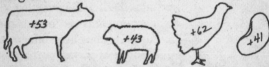

Liver stands head and shoulders above the other foods in this category. It is tremendously nutritious and terrifically well-rounded. A two-ounce serving of beef liver supplies the entire day's requirement for vitamin A and riboflavin. Beef liver gets 14 points for protein (28 percent of the RDA), 23 points for niacin (46 percent of the RDA), and 12 points for vitamin C (24 percent of the RDA); it is also credited with 14 points for iron and 5 points for being a good source of trace minerals. It loses only 3 points for its small content of fat. Some people increase the nutritional value of their hamburgers and meat loaf by grinding a quarter-pound of liver in with one pound of ground beef.

One objection that some people have to liver—

other than its taste—is that food contaminants, such as pesticides and hormones, may collect in that organ. Residues of the cancer-causing growth-hormone DES (diethylstilbestrol) that was fed to cattle were found almost exclusively in the liver. DES was outlawed by the Government in early 1973,* but other unsafe hormones, have replaced it. David Hawkins, an attorney with the Natural Resources Defense Council in Washington, D. C., has been at the forefront of the battle to keep animal drugs out of meat. Hawkins, and other attorneys and scientists like him, deserve the public's support. While they argue in the courts, however, the ranchers are feeding growth hormones to their cattle. The contamination of our food must be stopped, but until that is accomplished, I believe that the risk introduced by contaminants is outweighed by the well-balanced nutrition that liver offers. But eat only moderate amounts of liver, perhaps no more often than once or twice a month, unless you can find a store that sells organically raised meat.

Going quickly from the top to the bottom of the chart, we run into the worst of the meats: hot dog, bologna, bacon, and Spam. All of these contain lots of fat and relatively small amounts of protein, vitamins and minerals. They also contain the additive sodium nitrite, indicated by the asterisk, which should be avoided. Nitrite is hazardous because it can react with chemicals called amines in foods or drugs to produce nitrosamines. Extremely small amounts of nitrosamines have caused cancer in ani-

*FDA's ruling was overturned in court on a technicality, and DES was, at least temporarily, returned to use.

mals. U. S. Government chemists have found tiny amounts of nitrosamines in a number of samples of cured meats, with bacon containing more nitrosamines, more often, than any other food. Avoiding nitrite means avoiding cured meat: ham, liver sausage, bacon, hot dogs, bologna, salami, corned beef, etc. Nitrite is not necessary if a food is frozen, sterilized, or eaten soon after it is produced. A few health food stores and supermarkets sell nitrite-free hot dogs, bologna, and imitation bacon. Boycott nitrite-containing foods until the government bans nitrite. *Don't bring home the bacon!*

Americans have an almost insatiable desire for meat, particularly beef. In 1972, the average American devoured 116 pounds of beef, almost double the amount eaten as recently as 1950. In 1973, due to high prices, beef consumption dropped to 110 pounds per capita. This craving for beef means that we consume large amounts of saturated fat and cholesterol. Both of these substances tend to increase the amount of cholesterol in blood. This cholesterol can form plaques on the inner walls of blood vessels and make it difficult for the blood to pass. Eventually a blood clot may block the narrowed vessels and cause a heart attack or cerebral hemorrhage. Approximately half of all deaths is due to these two causes. Pot roast lost 12 points for fat content; roast ham had 14 points subtracted, sirloin steak 24 points.

Vegetable sources of protein, particularly soybeans, can be highly nutritious and are good substitutes for meat. Although kidney beans, black-eyed peas, navy beans, and pinto beans do not contain as high quality protein as meat and soybeans, they are also nourishing, especially when eaten with rice, corn, or a little meat. All grains and dried beans contain vitamins, minerals, some protein, fiber, very little fat, and no sugar. Many diet primarily on vegetable sources of protein instead of meat. Cooked with the right seasonings and sauces, beans and grains can be the basis of tempting, nutritious, inexpensive dishes. It might be interesting for you or your family to be vegetarians for a few days or a week. For recipe ideas, get a copy of *Recipes for a Small Planet* by Ellen Ewald.

Aside from benefiting your own health, eating more vegetable foods and less meat could help alleviate—in a small way—the world food problem. As Frances Moore Lappé describes so clearly in *Diet for a Small Planet*, American steers are usually fattened up on grains before slaughter. This is done partly because the Department of Agriculture's grading system (prime, choice, good) rewards carcasses that have a high fat content. Steers are very inefficient protein converters; for every twenty pounds of grain protein that they eat, they produce only about one pound of animal protein. This wastage borders on the criminal at a time when millions of persons are starving. This is not to say, though, that we must become vegetarians.

"In 1968 U.S. livestock (minus dairy cows) were fed 20 million tons of protein primarily from sources that could be eaten directly by man." Frances Moore Lappé, Diet for a Small Planet.

Cattle are very efficient at converting silage to meat and can graze on land that is too poor to grow crops. The public is going to have to pressure the Department of Agriculture, a bastion of conservatism, to promote more efficient ways of raising cattle. USDA should also be encouraging ranchers to raise breeds of cattle that are naturally low in fat.

SCOREBOARD 15

Protein Foods

FOOD	SERVING SIZE	NUTRITIONAL SCORE
Beef liver	2 oz.	172
Chicken liver	2 oz.	158
Liver sausage*	2 oz.	104
Chicken breast	2.7 oz.**	62
Tuna fish, packed in oil	3 oz.	55
Round steak, very lean	3 oz.	53
Turkey meat	3 oz.	52
Sockeye salmon, canned	3 oz.	48
Pork chop, lean	1.7 oz.**	47
Hamburger, lean	3 oz.	46
Veal cutlet	3 oz.	45
Round steak, lean and fat	3 oz.	43
Lamb chop, lean	2.6 oz.**	43
Leg of lamb, lean, roasted	2½ oz.	43
Soybeans, cooked	½ cup	41
Cod, broiled	3 oz.	40

Food	Serving Size	Nutritional Score
Flounder, baked	3 oz.	38
Eggs	2	36
Roast ham, lean and fat*	3 oz.	35
Hamburger, regular	3 oz.	34
Pot roast, lean and fat	3 oz.	33
Navy beans	½ cup	32
Alpo dog food (fortified)	3 oz.	30
Pork chop, lean and fat	1.7 oz.**	29
Salami*	2 oz. (2 slices)	27
Pork sausage	2 oz. (2 links)	27
Drumstick, chicken, fried	1.3 oz.**	26
Lentils, cooked	½ cup	24
Shrimp	1½ oz.	24
Ham, boiled and sliced*	2 oz.	22
Sirloin steak, lean and fat	3 oz.	19
McDonald's small hamburger	1.6 oz.	18
Peanut butter	2 Tbsp.	17
Hot dog, pure beef*	1	6
Spam*	3 oz.	4
Bacon*	3 slices	4
Bologna*	2 oz. (2 slices)	2

*These foods contain sodium nitrite, an additive that should be avoided.
**Weight does not include the bone.

Bread, Rice, and Pasta

One of the recurring questions about foods is "which is better, whole wheat bread or enriched white bread?" White flour, which is used to make white bread, cakes, and rolls, consists largely of the least nutritious part of the wheat berry, the starchy endosperm (see Figure 4). The wheat germ, which is a rich source of vitamins and minerals, and the bran, which contains nutrients and fiber, are both selectively removed in the milling process and used in animal feed. Plain white flour is a nutritional disaster. White flour that is enriched by the addition of several of the vitamins and minerals that are lost in milling is a clear improvement. However, many of the lost nutrients are not replaced.

The Food and Nutrition Board of the National Academy of Sciences issued a report in 1974 that recommended the addition of ten vitamins and minerals to white flour (it is now fortified with four or five nutrients). But the Board acknowledged that even this expanded fortification effort would not make white flour equivalent to whole wheat flour. The report said:

Because of the increasing recognition of the importance

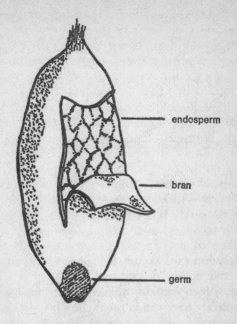

endosperm

bran

germ

A Wheat Berry

of certain of these trace nutrients in our diets today, it is urged that processors of wheat, in the interest of retaining the maximum amount of all nutrients indigenous to wheat, refine flour no more than is actually required for consumer acceptance and that they avoid the use of destructive bleaching and maturing agents wherever possible.[80]

Consumers can encourage bread manufacturers to follow this advice by buying whole wheat bread.

The FDA has recognized that enriching foods with nutrients is a practical way, but not the ideal way of providing good nutrition. In 1943 FDA said that " ... adequate nutrition could be better assured through the choice of natural foods than through reliance on enrichment...." FDA concluded, though, that the nourishing natural foods were not always available and that most consumers did not know enough about nutrition to choose a well-rounded diet from un-enriched natural foods.[80]

Because white bread is fortified with several nutrients that our formula considers, it receives more points than whole wheat bread for riboflavin (6 vs. 1.7), niacin (4.3 vs. 3.6), and iron (4 vs. 3.1). Whole wheat bread contains more magnesium (5 vs. 1), pyridoxine (2 vs. 0.5), fiber (1.6 vs. 0.2), and trace minerals (2.6 vs. 0) than does enriched white bread. In addition, whole wheat bread is a richer source of certain other vitamins and minerals, such as folic acid and pantothenic acid, that are not factors in the rating system.

The one possible problem with whole wheat bread is that it contains phytic acid, while white bread has relatively little. Phytic acid is the storage form of phosphorus in wheat. As the grain germinates, the phytic acid is broken down to release phosphate, which is used by the plant for growth. Phytate in the diet can be a problem, because it combines with calcium, zinc, and possibly other minerals, reducing their availability to the body. In some Middle East villages, dwarfism due to zinc deficiency is common. The zinc deficiency is thought to be due to diets that consist primarily of unleavened whole wheat bread, which is high in phytic acid. Most Americans obtain only about 10-20 percent of their calories from grains, and so any adverse effects of phytic acid would be minimal.

Furthermore, according to Dr. Jean Mayer, much of the phytic acid is destroyed in the leavening process. However, those few persons whose diets are based to a much larger extent on whole grain foods should also eat non-grain foods that are rich in zinc and other trace minerals (meat, liver, eggs, shellfish, fish). Dr. Mayer, after weighing the arguments about phytic acid, concluded that "in this country, phytate should not be considered a serious impediment to the process of metabolizing calcium, especially if you eat a well-balanced diet."[81]

Enriched white bread contains more iron and several B-vitamins than whole wheat bread, but in most other respects whole wheat bread is superior. On balance, as the Scoreboard shows, whole wheat bread with a score of 26 is more nutritious than enriched white bread with a score of 22. The difference in scores would be even greater, but for the fact that the nutrients added to white bread are some of the very ones that are considered in our rating formula. Make every effort to eat more whole wheat bread, rolls, and pancakes, and less white bread and other foods made with enriched (or non-enriched) white flour. And don't overlook rye bread, which heads Scoreboard 16.

Shoppers should be aware that bakers often use artificial coloring to make a loaf of bread look more nutritious than it really is. Some dark, nutritious-looking breads are little more than white breads in disguise. Bakers add caramel coloring to pumpernickel, "wheat bread" (all bread is made from wheat), and rye bread to make them look as if they contain more whole grain flour than they really do. In the old days, egg bread and butter-

and-egg bread were yellow, because of their egg or butter content. Bakers, however, now add yellow food coloring to mask the fact that they use so little butter and so few eggs. The Center for Science in the Public Interest and Professor Donald Davis (then at the University of California, Irvine) petitioned FDA in June, 1974, to put a halt to these blatant examples of adulteration, but FDA rejected the petition in June, 1975. So it's still *Caveat emptor* . . . be sure to read your labels carefully.

The story of rice is similar to that of bread. Brown rice contains all the nutritive value of a rice grain. Most Americans, however, prefer the taste, texture, and color of the white rice which is left after the nutrient-rich bran and germ are removed in milling. White rice is usually enriched, which means that a few of the nutrients (B-vitamins and iron) lost in milling are restored. A more nutritious form of white rice is the parboiled or converted variety. It is made by heating whole rice in such a way that some of the nutrients migrate from the outer parts of the grain—which are later lost in milling—to the part of the grain that is saved. If you have never tried brown rice, buy a pound of the long grain variety and give your taste buds a new experience.

Spaghetti and macaroni are ordinarily made with refined flour, but you may be able to get whole wheat pasta from a local natural foods store. Whole wheat pasta is better than regular pasta for the same reasons that whole wheat bread is better than white bread.

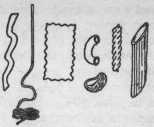

Bread, rice, and pasta have gotten an ill-deserved reputation of being high in calories and low in nutrients. In fact, whole grains are quite well-balanced foods. They are not especially high in calories, and the fiber helps create a feeling of fullness. Most people in the world base their diet to a great extent on rice and wheat (and are usually quite healthy if they get enough calories). Most Americans consume far too much fat for our own good, and somewhat too much protein. To reduce our intake of these nutrients, we will have to consume more carbohydrate-rich foods. Whole wheat bread, brown rice, bulghur wheat, and other whole grain foods are excellent foods and should be eaten routinely. They are also among the least expensive foods.

SCOREBOARD 16

Bread, Rice, and Pasta

FOOD	SERVING SIZE	NUTRITIONAL SCORE
Breads		
Rye bread (American)	2 slices	29
Whole wheat bread	2 slices	26
Pumpernickel bread	2 slices	26
White bread, enriched	2 slices	22
Hamburger or hot dog bun	1	18
White bread, not enriched	2 slices	12
Rice		
Brown rice	½ cup	22
Parboiled rice	½ cup	17
White rice, enriched	½ cup	16
Instant rice, enriched	½ cup	14
Pasta		
Egg noodles, enriched	0.9 cup*	28
Elbow macaroni, enriched	¾ cup*	26
Spaghetti, enriched	¾ cup*	26
Crackers		
Triscuit crackers	4 (.6 oz.)	9
Saltines	4 (.4 oz.)	8

*One ounce before cooking.

Frozen and Canned
Prepared Meals

In the last twenty years frozen, dehydrated, and canned dinners have changed from bad jokes to, in some cases, tasty and nourishing meals. Aside from taste, the worst things about many of these products were the petite portions and lack of nutritional balance. Companies have begun to meet

> **A meal is more than food:** "The simple fact is that practically nowhere in this country do people of different age groups sit down to meals together anymore. That, of course, means they simply don't communicate with each other . . . Most of us do still think of meals as deeply significant in bringing people closer together. Just the same, family meals are disappearing . . . Food technology is a great thing, but we must not let it destroy mealtimes and, with them, a bridge between generations." Dr. Jean Mayer, Professor of Nutrition, Harvard School of Public Health, 1973.

these objections, though, by introducing "Hungry Man" and similar large-sized dinners. Some companies have also been able to crash through the taste barrier.

Scoreboard 17 lists just a few of the scores of frozen or canned whole-meal products that are available at supermarkets. Note that the sizes of the products vary over a considerable range. The scores are comparatively high, because they represent a whole meal, rather than a single food.

In order to have a complete, well-rounded meal, most of these products should be eaten with bread and spread, a glass of milk or juice, and a nutritious dessert.

SCOREBOARD 17

Frozen and Canned Prepared Meals

FOOD	SERVING SIZE	NUTRITIONAL SCORE
Morton sliced turkey dinner	17 oz.	144
Swanson beef deep dish pie	16 oz.	142
Morton meat loaf dinner	17 oz.	141
Swanson turkey deep dish pie	16 oz.	139
Morton sliced beef dinner	17 oz.	136
Swanson ham TV dinner*		131

Food	Serving Size	Nutritional Score
Swanson chicken deep dish pie	16 oz.	129
Morton chicken and dumplings	17 oz.	127
Morton salisbury steak dinner	17 oz.	125
Swanson fried chicken TV dinner		125
Swanson 3-course fried chicken dinner	15.5 oz.	118
Swanson 3-course meat loaf dinner		113
Swanson 3-course turkey dinner	16 oz.	108
Swanson 3-course salisbury steak dinner		104
Swanson veal parmigiana TV dinner	12.25 oz.	96
Morton fried chicken dinner	17 oz.	93
Swanson turkey TV dinner	11.5 oz.	89
Swanson filet of ocean fish TV dinner		84
Bounty beef stew	1 cup	84
Swanson spaghetti and meatballs TV dinner		80
Morton macaroni and cheese dinner	10 oz.	79
Bounty chicken stew	1 cup	77

Food	Serving Size	Nutritional Score
Swanson chopped sirloin beef TV dinner	10 oz.	76
Pork and beans	1 cup	70
Swanson meat loaf TV dinner		67
Bounty chili con carne with beans	1 cup	65
Swanson chicken pot pie	8 oz.	64
Dinty Moore beef stew	8 oz.	61
Swanson beef pot pie	8 oz.	60
Swanson turkey pot pie	8 oz.	58
Swanson beans and franks TV dinner*		57
Franco-American spaghetti	1 cup	55
Franco-American spaghetti and meatballs in tomato sauce	1 cup	50
Franco-American macaroni and cheese	1 cup	44
Hunt-Wesson Manwich, regular	1/6 can	43

*These foods contain sodium nitrite, an additive that should be avoided.

Breakfast Foods

In 1970 Robert Choate sent shock waves through America's kitchens by testifying at a Senate hearing about the nutritional deficiencies of breakfast cereals. Americans were startled to learn that some of their favorite foods were sugar-coated nutritional nothings. In the past three years the major breakfast cereal producers have responded to the adverse publicity by producing a few new cereals (some good, some bad), and by spraying most of their products with vitamins. As things now stand, the breakfast cereal market as a whole is not much better than it was in 1970. A few products—Puffed Wheat and Puffed Rice—are little more than starch and air. At the other extreme, some products—Product 19, Concentrate, Kaboom, Total, and King Vitaman—have been sprayed with so many vitamins and minerals that they are as much vitamin pills as breakfast cereals. Many popular cereals—Sugar Frosted Flakes, Kaboom, Super Sugar Crisp—are heavily fortified with nutrients, but in addition contain so much sugar that they would be better called breakfast candy. In fact, a 1974 statement by the

Food and Nutrition Board of the National Research Council said that sugar-coated cereals "do not contain sufficient cereal to warrant their classification as a breakfast cereal. They more properly belong in the category of snack foods. ..." Finally, a few cereals remain that are not overly sugared, not sprayed with vitamins, and not overly processed: oatmeal, wheat germ, shredded wheat, granola, and Familia.

Because manufacturers can spray whatever they make with inexpensive nutrients, cereals listed on the Scoreboard were ranked according to sugar content rather than nutritional value. If the cereal contains gobs of sugar, avoid it, regardless of how many nutrients it has been coated with. Sugar-coated cereals may account for 10 to 15 percent of a child's daily sugar intake (assuming two one-ounce servings a day). These cereals, especially when eaten as snacks, contribute to tooth decay. Avoid also the cereals that are sprayed with artificial coloring. Coloring adds to the cost and subtracts from the safety; it does not add to the nutritional value. Most of the colored cereals—Franken-Berry, Alpha-Bits, Kaboom, etc.—contain 30-45 percent sugar.

After you exclude the highly sweetened and colored cereals, you are on your own. You can buy a fortified product or you can stick to the "natural" cereals. Wheat germ is probably the best of the naturals, because it consists entirely of the most nutritious part of the wheat berry. Shredded wheat, granola, and oatmeal are also whole grain cereals. All-Bran is the best source of dietary fiber. If you buy a fortified product, you could be paying dearly for vitamins you may not need. For instance, one of the biggest gyps in the marketplace is General Mills' (the Big G) Total. Total is the same as Wheaties—also made by the Big G—except that it has been sprayed with one-half-cents-worth more vitamins (12-ounce box). At the store you pay about 26 cents more for that half-cent's worth of vitamins. Total is one reason why some people say that the Big G stands for the Big Gyp. A six-year-old child who eats two one-ounce servings of Total would get four times as much vitamin A as it needed for the whole day.

The hottest new sellers in the cereal market are the new "natural" cereals, like Quaker 100% Natural, Alpen, and Kellogg's Country Morning. Far from being innovations, these products are actually just well-packaged, higher-priced versions of cereals that have been sold for years in health food stores. They are good in that they represent a tacit admission by the food industry that "natural" foods still do have a place in the supermarket, along with all the processed novelties. They are also made largely from whole grains, nuts, and seeds. Unfortunately, however, the cereal corporations are so

"Recent research indicates that more and more mothers everywhere are aware of the need for vitamin and mineral fortification. And are even willing to pay a little extra for it . . . we can show you why it pays to fortify." Roche Chemical Division, Hoffman-La Roche, Inc., 1971.

used to coating everything with sugar that they have added large amounts of sugar to most of the so-called natural cereals. Quaker's 100% Natural is approximately one-fifth sugar, and should really be called Quaker 80% Natural. The rule still holds; avoid sugar-coated cereals, even ones made with whole grains.

Shopping is made immeasurably more confusing by the vast array of breakfast cereals with which we are faced. Companies have been engaged in a great War for Shelf-space. They began producing every variety of cereal their chemists and advertising agents could think of. Total is nothing but heavily fortified Wheaties. Trix is nothing but colored and sweetened Kix. The impetus for the War for Shelf-space was that companies realized that the cereal market is a flexible and impulsive one. The greater the number of company X's cereals on a supermarket shelf, the greater the likelihood that the shopper will select a company X product.

Of course, another reason for all the new sugary cereals is television. Cereal companies saw television for what it is: a salesperson that can reach into every home and persuade the children to make Mommy buy a certain product. Ad agents and technologists then devised products that were specially geared to the child market and mentality. Most of these products are loaded with sugar and coloring. The same concern for our children's welfare that condemns dope pushers in the playground should also demand that junk dealers be banished from the TV screen in the living room.

Action for Children's Television (ACT, Newtonville, Mass. 02160) has been at the forefront of the battle to ban advertising aimed at children. ACT, which was started in 1968 by several concerned mothers, is a marvelous example of how ordinary citizens can form influential organizations. As a direct result of ACT's work, stations are reducing the amount of advertising on children's programs (from sixteen minutes per hour down to nine and a half by the end of 1975). Furthermore, commercials for vitamin pills have been completely dropped from "kidvid," as it is called in the trade. ACT is now aiming its sights at sugar-rich foods, including cereals.

In August, 1974, health professionals joined the attack on sugar-coated cereals. More than 600 nutritionists, dentists, dietitians, doctors, and nutrition students, along with twenty-two citizens groups and professional associations, petitioned FDA to set a "standard of quality" for breakfast cereals. Cereals containing less than 10 percent sugar could be marketed as they are. But products containing more than 10 percent sugar would have to bear a label statement reading: "Contains—% Sugar; Frequent Use Contributes to Tooth Decay and Other Health Problems." Endorsers of the petition, which was circulated by Center for Science in the Public Interest, included Dr. Jean Mayer (Harvard School of Public Health), Drs. George Briggs and Doris Calloway (University of California, Berkeley), Action for Children's Television, American Public Health Association, and American Society for Preventive Dentistry.

The petition quoted FDA Assistant Commissioner Dr. Lloyd Tepper, who at a 1973 Senate

Hearing criticized sugar-coated cereals. Dr. Tepper said:

I don't think you have to be a great scientist to appreciate the fact that a highly sweetened, sucrose-containing material, which is naturally tacky when it gets wet, is going to be a troublemaker. And I would not prescribe this particular food component for my own children, not on the basis of scientific studies, but because I do not believe that prolonged exposure of tooth surfaces to a sucrose-containing material of this sort is beneficial.[82]

The FDA denied the petition, but the fight to clean up the breakfast cereal market is far from over.

☞ How to Choose a Cereal ☜

The best way to judge the quality of a breakfast cereal is to read carefully the list of ingredients on the label. If sugar is listed first, avoid the product, regardless of how many nutrients have been added. Select cereals that contain whole grains and little or no sugar. Here are two labels:

Wheatena
INGREDIENTS
100% natural wheat. Contains no added salt or any other additives or preservatives.

FRANKEN•BERRY
INGREDIENTS
Sugar, oat flour, degermed yellow corn meal, wheat and corn starch, corn syrup, dextrose, salt, gelatin, coconut and peanut oils, calcium carbonate, sodium phosphate, monoglycerides, artificial flavors, sodium ascorbate, artificial colors, niacin, iron, gum acacia, vitamin A palmitate, pyridoxine (vitamin B_6), riboflavin, thiamin, vitamin D and vitamin B_{12}. Freshness preserved by BHT.

What's wrong with Franken·Berry?

1) Sugar is listed first, which means that it is the major ingredient. The cereal also contains two other sweeteners, corn syrup and dextrose, which add calories without nutrients.
2) It contains starch, refined, and degermed flour instead of whole-grain flour.
3) It contains artificial colors, artificial flavors, and the artificial preservative BHT.

What's right with Wheatena? It is made with whole wheat and does not contain added sugar or artificial coloring. It is also relatively inexpensive, 63¢ for 22 ounces (2.9¢ per ounce) compared to 65¢ for 8 ounces (8.1¢ per ounce) of Franken·Berry.

Cost of Breakfast Cereals

Kellogg's Corn Flakes
   12 ounce box   45¢   3.75¢ per ounce

Kellogg's Sugar Frosted Flakes
   10 ounce box   55¢   5.5¢ per ounce

You pay almost twice as much for sugar-coated corn flakes as for plain, old-fashioned corn flakes. You pay extra for a product that is not as good for your body.

While sugar-coated cereals are unwholesome

foods, we should remember that they are certainly not the only foods that contribute to our high intake of sugar. The average person, for instance, consumes far more sugar from soda pop than from cereals. Cereals, however, in their large and brightly colored boxes, have come to symbolize the deterioration of our food supply. Reducing the sugar levels in cereals would make a small contribution to health. It would also do much to establish a climate for eliminating other junk foods.

Breakfast foods are listed in Scoreboard 18. This Scoreboard differs from the others in that the foods are ranked in order of sugar content, rather than nutritional score. This is done because the points that some cereals gain from added vitamins and iron completely obscure the points lost due to a high sugar content. If the products were ranked according to score, King Vitaman would be third on the list, despite being docked 35 points for its high sugar content. Remember, vitamins and minerals that are added to foods do increase the nutritional value of the foods, but do not cancel out the detrimental effects of high sugar or fat contents.

Breakfast can be a psychedelic experience. Don't believe for a minute that your menu must be limited to bacon and eggs or breakfast cereals. Many of us have come to think that eating anything but a packaged cereal would violate the U.S. Constitution. Breakfast can be a time to use up some of the leftovers in the refrigerator. Have some chicken; a cold, boiled potato; peas and carrots; grapefruit or watermelon. Dip into the fruit and vegetable bins. Or make a toasted cheese or peanut butter or tuna sandwich on whole wheat bread. Pour a glass of orange juice and a glass of milk. Start the day with a hearty, wholesome, different kind of breakfast, and the sun may seem a little brighter, the sky a little bluer.

SCOREBOARD 18
Breakfast Foods
(1 oz. portion unless stated otherwise)

FOOD	PERCENTAGE SUGAR**
Cream of Wheat (50)*	0
Wheat germ (48)	0
Granola, made with honey (25)	0
Shredded wheat, 1 biscuit (22)	0
Oatmeal, ⅔ cup (20)	0
Farina, ⅔ cup (18)	0
Puffed wheat, ½ oz. (13)	0
Puffed rice, ½ oz. (5)	0
Cheerios (75)	4
Rice Chex (62)	5
Wheat Chex (84)	6
Raisin bran (96)	6
Rice Krispies (62)	7
Kellogg's corn flakes (61)	7
Post Toasties (61)	7
Special K (73)	9
Total (189)	11
Kellogg's Concentrate (95)	11
Wheaties (75)	11
Product 19 (176)	12
Alpen***	13

Food	Percentage Sugar**
Life (64)	14
Corn Chex (56)	14
Quaker 100% Natural (5)	19
Fortified Oat Flakes (84)	20
Pop Tart	26
Sugar Frosted Flakes (44)	29
Super Sugar Chex (8)	33
Cap'n Crunch (26)	37
Cocoa Krispies (38)	38
Alpha Bits (38)	40
Super Sugar Crisp (34)	43
Fruity or Cocoa Pebbles (33)	44
King Vitaman (161)	50

*Most cereals are fortified with vitamins and minerals. The number in parentheses is the nutritional rating.

**Calculated by the author; all companies refused to disclose the sugar content of their products.

***Not calculated.

Snacks

Eleven o'clock in the morning, you get the hungries and crave a snack. The kids come home from school, take off their coats and ask for a snack. Sitting up late watching the tube, the stomach rumbles and you reach for a snack. Snacks are making up a bigger and bigger part of our diet and the food producers recognize this. Not only have they responded by producing a mind-boggling variety of products—ranging from bite-size candies to Screaming Yellow Zonkers and Fiddle Faddles—but they have packaged them in single-serving portions for vending machines, which are everywhere. Unfortunately, most of the commercial snacks are nutritional abominations: high in sugar, high in saturated fat, high in salt; low in vitamins, low in minerals, low in protein.

Snacks do not have to be junk. As Scoreboard 19 shows, a handful of nuts has a score ranging from 17 for walnuts to 25 for peanuts and 31 for almonds. One-quarter cup of sunflower seeds scores 44 points. When you buy nuts and seeds, try to get them without all the salt.

Apples and peaches are great snacks any time.

Both contain fiber and Vitamin C; in addition, peaches contain vitamin A. Raisins contain iron, but consist largely of sugar that can stick between teeth and promote tooth decay.

For the late night snacks, have a bowl of granola with milk—it is exceptionally satisfying and offers well-balanced nutrition. Popcorn is OK, at least until it is coated with butter and sprinkled with salt; after all, popcorn is whole kernel corn. The worst thing you can do to popcorn is soak it in sugary syrup, which is basically what Cracker Jack is. The nutritional rating for Cracker Jack is −39 because of all the sugar. The score would be even lower were it not for the peanuts they throw in, which contribute some vitamins, minerals, and protein. But, of course, if you want peanuts, don't buy Cracker Jack, buy peanuts.

Candy bars contain a considerable amount of sugar and oil and have the low scores that we would expect. Not all candy bars are the same, as the Scoreboard shows, although all have negative scores. Among the candy bars that Mars makes, 3-Muskateers is the worst, with a rating of −55, and Snickers is the best. Snickers has a decent amount of protein (5 points), niacin (5 points), and cal-

"[Food manufacturers] are absolutely convinced that for the pre-puberty set, sugar appeal is the counterpart of sex appeal." Robert Choate, Council on Children, Media, and Merchandising, 1972.

cium (3 points), which come from the milk, peanuts, egg whites, and vegetable protein. The sugar (−37 points) and oil (−8 points) more than offset the good ingredients in Snickers. The standard 1½-ounce package of Chuckles contains 150 calories—this is almost 10 percent of one's daily caloric intake!

As Scoreboard 19 indicates, a Hostess Sno-Ball has a pretty abysmal score (−44). This score is low despite the fact that the manufacturer, ITT-Continental Baking, spikes the product with vitamins and iron and proclaims *vitamin fortified* on the wrapper. The Sno-Ball loses 53 points because of its enormous sugar content. You can do with the Hostess Sno-Ball what you do with a real snowball: throw it away as far and as fast as you can.

Snacking on sugar-containing foods is the quickest way to develop tooth decay. The classic study demonstrating this was conducted twenty-five years ago on patients in a mental hospital in Vipeholm, Sweden.[83] This carefully controlled study showed that eating sugary foods frequently between meals causes much more tooth decay than eating the same foods only at meals. If you care about your teeth (and if you don't care about your own teeth, what do you care about?), eat snacks that do not contain sugar and indulge your sweet tooth only at mealtimes. Why pay for your dentist's trip to Bermuda?

There is nothing wrong with eating between meals. Many doctors even recommend lots of little meals in place of three big ones. But it is easy to fall into the habit of eating junky snacks that push more nutritious foods out of our diet, contribute to

183

tooth decay, and add on the pounds. Try to keep a variety of nutritious snacks around the house, school, cafeteria, clubhouse, or office. Ditto for parties—don't feel compelled to buy the junky "party" foods that smile down from supermarket shelves. Nuts, roasted soybeans, cheese, raw broccoli and cauliflower, and fruit are convenient, nutritious, delicious, and fun to eat.

SCOREBOARD 19

Snacks

Food	Serving Size	Nutritional Score
Granola and milk	1 oz. plus ½ cup	45
Sunflower seeds	¼ cup	44
Almonds	¼ cup	31
Peach	1	29
Peanuts	¼ cup	25
Granola	1 oz.	25
Cashews	¼ cup	24
Walnuts	¼ cup	17
Raisins	1½ oz.	13
Apple	1	12
Triscuit crackers	4 (0.6 oz.)	9
Potato chips	¾ oz.	8
Popcorn (no butter)	2 cups	6
Oatmeal cookie	1	− 4
Sandwich cookie	1	− 7
Snickers candy	1 bar	−23

Food	Serving Size	Nutritional Score
Mar's Almond candy	1 bar	−27
Milk chocolate	1 oz.	−27
Brownie	1 (1⅛ oz.)	−30
Milky Way candy	1 bar	−33
M & M's candy	1 pack	−33
Cracker Jack	1 box	−39
Hostess Sno-Ball	1	−44
Popsicle	1 (3 oz.)	−45
3-Musketeers candy	1 bar	−55
Chuckles candy	1 package	−74

Desserts

After a delicious, hearty meal our taste buds often yearn for a bit of sweetness, a dessert, to add the crowning touch to a pleasurable experience. The dessert is usually the weakest part of the meal as far as nutrition goes, and this is nothing new. Sugar-rich cakes, pies, ice cream, and cookies have been traditional desserts for generations. As Scoreboard 20 shows, though, with some care we can greatly improve the nutritional value of our desserts and still please our taste buds. In many homes an after-dinner fruit bowl is a tradition. A peach, apple, or banana is a way of getting sweetness along with some vitamins and minerals. Two of the tastiest treats—cantaloupe with a small scoop of ice cream, and a cold wedge of watermelon—are also among the most nutritious.

Canned fruit is especially nutritious and wholesome when it is packed in juice or water, but usually it is packed in a thick sugar syrup. The rating of peaches canned in water is 16, but the rating of peaches in heavy syrup is —24. Heavy syrup reduces the rating of pineapple from 27 to 4. Unsweetened applesauce scores 9, but the sweetened variety scores —35.

Many of the commercial products that are sold as desserts are nutritional disasters. Morton coconut pie, those flip-top cans of imitation pudding, and gelatin desserts contain little besides sugar, water, oil, artificial coloring and flavoring, and a flock of chemical additives to hold them together. Jell-O and other gelatin desserts, despite

"The consumption of sugar and other relatively pure carbohydrates has become so great during recent years that it presents a serious obstacle to the improved nutrition of the general public." Council on Foods and Nutrition, American Medical Association, 1942.

their longstanding place in the market, are among the worst foods. They are mainly sugar, and contain artificial coloring and artificial flavoring. They do contain a little of the protein "gelatin," but it is of such low quality that it is almost useless to the body. All in all, a gelatin dessert has no redeeming nutritional value and certainly deserves its score of —45 for a ½-cup serving.

It is not just store-bought desserts that have low ratings. Homemade brownies, chocolate cake, and apple pie also have disaster-zone scores, because they contain so much sugar. It is from products like these that so much sugar and other refined sweeteners (126 pounds per year per person) sneak into our diet. However, if we substitute whole wheat flour for white flour and use less sugar, homemade desserts can be much more nutritious than Betty Crocker's.

SCOREBOARD 20

Desserts

FOOD	SERVING SIZE	NUTRITIONAL SCORE
Cantaloupe with ice cream	¼ melon, 1½ oz. ice cream	90
Watermelon	2 lbs.*	74
Peach	1	29
Pineapple, canned in juice	½ cup	27
Peaches, canned, water pack	½ cup	16
Apple	1	12

Food	Serving Size	Nutritional Score
Applesauce, unsweetened	½ cup	9
Pineapple, canned in heavy syrup	½ cup	4
Blueberry muffin	1 (1⅛ oz.)	0
Peaches, canned in light syrup	½ cup	− 6
Angel food cake	1/12 cake (2 oz.)	−15
Cool 'n Creamy	½ cup	−18
Ice cream	3 oz.	−18
Hunt Snack Pack fruit cup	1	−19
Hunt Snack Pack vanilla pudding	1	−20
Peaches, canned in heavy syrup	½ cup	−24
Coconut	1½ oz.	−30
Brownie	1 (1⅛ oz.)	−30
Applesauce, sweetened	½ cup	−35
Apple pie	6 oz.	−40
Del Monte vanilla pudding	1	−43
Jell-O	½ cup	−45
Chocolate cake	3 oz.	−52
Morton coconut cream pie	¼ pie	−62
Ice cream soda	8 oz. soda; 3 oz. ice cream	−79

*This weight includes the rind; however, any nutrients in the rind were not included in the score.

Odds and Ends

Remember, you can add the ratings of individual foods to determine the score of a "compound food," like a sandwich. This Scoreboard will help you determine the scores of such items as a hamburger with catsup or french fries with mayonnaise.

An easy way of adding to the taste and nutritional value of your food is to sprinkle wheat germ on ice cream and in breakfast cereals or to add it to meat loaf and hamburgers. Wheat germ is an especially good source of thiamin and trace minerals.

Catsup, which consists primarily of tomatoes, contains small amounts of vitamins A and C. Catsup's score of 2 for one tablespoon would be significantly higher if some of the vitamin C were not destroyed in processing or if it did not contain sugar. The presence of perhaps 10 percent sugar in catsup is one of many ways that sugar has snuck into our diet. Sugar may be present in catsup without being listed on the label.

A couple of foods on this chart reveal some of the limitations of the food rating system. Honey has a positive score of 3 (from carbohydrate and

HOW DOES YOUR DIET RATE?

FOOD	SERVING	SCORE
Breakfast		
Mid-morning		
Lunch		
Afternoon		
Dinner		
After dinner		
	total	

Make extra copies of charts like this on other sheets of paper.

B-vitamins), which would indicate that it is fairly nutritious. In fact, however, honey is over 80 percent sugar and is basically empty calories. It contains trivial amounts of vitamins and minerals. Honey makes foods sticky and can contribute to tooth decay. Aside from its taste, the best thing about honey (to those kill-joy nutritionists) is its high price—this keeps people from eating too much of it. The average consumption of honey in the U.S. is only one pound per person per year, as compared to over one hundred pounds of sugar.

Mayonnaise has a low score, −7, although it contains polyunsaturated vegetable oil. Recall that our formula penalizes foods if more than 36 percent of their calories come from fat or oil. Ninety-eight percent of the calories in mayonnaise come from the oil, and the points lost for this more than balance the credit received for having polyunsaturated oil. Americans receive 40 to 50 percent of their calories from fats, as compared to the recommended 20 to 35 percent.

The items at the very bottom of Scoreboard 21 contain large amounts of sugar. Remember syrup's ignoble position, anchoring the chart, before pouring it on your (whole wheat) pancakes next Sunday. Use berries or margarine instead.

SCOREBOARD 24

Odds and Ends

Food	Serving Size	Nutritional Score
Wheat germ	1 Tbsp.	10
Honey	1 Tbsp.	3
Catsup	1 Tbsp.	2
Cream	¾ oz.	1
Margarine, soft (made with liquid oil)	1 pat	0
Margarine, regular	1 pat	− 1
Butter	1 pat	− 3
Cool Whip	1 Tbsp.	− 4
Salad dressing	1 Tbsp.	− 4
Coffee whitener (made with coconut oil)	¾ oz.	− 5
Mayonnaise	1 Tbsp.	− 7
Butter	1 Tbsp.	− 9
Jelly	1 Tbsp.	− 9
Sugar	1 tsp.	− 9
Sugar	1 Tbsp.	−27
Syrup	1 Tbsp.	−34

Sample Diets

A Nutrition-conscious Person

FOOD		SERVING	CALORIES	FOOD RATING
Breakfast:	Wheat Chex	1 oz.	120	84
	Skim Milk	8 oz.	90	49
	Grapefruit	½	45	45
	Coffee	8 oz.	3	0
Snack:	Peach	1	35	29
Lunch:	Creamed Cottage Cheese with	1 cup	260	
	Tomato	1	40	69
	Whole-Wheat Bread with	1 slice	62	13
	Swiss Cheese	2 oz.	200	43
	Iced Tea	8 oz.	3	0
Snack:	Peanuts	¼ cup	210	25
Dinner:	Chicken Breast	2.7 oz. (no bone)	155	62
	Broccoli	3⅛ oz.	26	116
	Enriched Egg Noodles	.9 oz.	164	28
	Skim Milk	8 oz.	90	49
	Fruit Salad:			
	Strawberries	½ cup	28	50
	Cantaloupe	¼ melon	45	99
	Raisins	1½ oz.	82	13
			1658	842

A Food Faddist

FOOD		SERVING	CALORIES	FOOD RATING
Breakfast:	Cocoa Krispies	1 oz.	111	38
	Whole Milk	4 oz.	160	19
	Pop Tarts	2	416	42
Snack:	Cracker Jack	1 box	75	−39
Lunch:	Hot Dog	1	142	6
	and Bun	1	114	18
	Potato Chips	¾ oz.	115	8
	Hunts Snack Pack			
	Pudding	1	238	−20
	Hi-C	6 oz.	89	4
Snack:	Ice Cream	3 oz.	95	−18
	Mom's Apple Pie	6 oz.	243	−10
	Soda Pop	12 oz.	145	−12
Dinner:	Swanson Spaghetti			
	and Meatball			
	TV Dinner	1	323	80
	Soda Pop	12 oz.	145	−92
	Chocolate Cake	3 oz.	338	−53
Snack:	Snickers Candy			
	Bar	1	240	−23
	Soda Pop	12 oz.	145	−92
			3134	−254

Appendix 1

*1973 Advertising Budgets of Major Food Producers**

General Foods	$180,000,000	8.1% of sales
Heublein Inc. (Kentucky Fried Chicken, Smirnoff vodka)	77,800,000	5.9%
Coca Cola Co.	76,000,000	3.5%
General Mills	74,200,000	3.7%
Kraftco Corp. (cheeses)	74,000,000	2.4%
Nabisco	69,050,000	6.8%
Distillers Corp.—Seagrams	65,192,000	3.9%
Norton Simon, Inc. (Wesson, Hunt)	61,700,000	5.1%
PepsiCo	58,000,000	4.4%
Pillsbury Co.	50,000,000	5.0%
Standard Brands, Inc. (Planter's, Fleischmann)	50,000,000	4.5%
McDonald's Corp.	46,500,000	3.1%
Kellogg Co.	45,000,000	5.4%
Campbell Soup Co.	40,000,000	3.7%
Ralston Purina Co.	38,500,000	1.6%
Anheuser Busch, Inc.	36,520,000	2.5%
Jos. Schlitz Brewing Co.	34,500,000	3.9%

*Estimates taken from *Advertising Age*, August 26, 1974, reprinted with permission.

CPC International (Skippy, Hellmann's)	34,200,000	4.0%
Wm. Wrigley Jr. Co.	28,100,000	12.1%
Thomas Lipton Inc.	28,000,000	6.9%
Seven-Up Co.	27,358,000	18.6%
Nestle Co.	27,000,000	4.5%
H. J. Heinz Co.	26,000,000	1.8%
Quaker Oats Co.	26,000,000	2.6%
National Distillers & Chem. (Almaden wine, whiskey)	23,500,000	1.9%
Hiram Walker (whiskey)	23,000,000	2.7%
Carnation Co.	21,000,000	1.4%
Mars Inc. (candy)	19,000,000	12.3%

Appendix 2

Food and Drug Administration

Peter Hutt, General Counsel	came from	Covington & Burling law firm; represented ITT-Continental Baking Milk Industry Foundation, Institute of Shortening and Edible Oils, and many other firms
William Goodrich, General Counsel	went to	President, Institute of Shortening and Edible Oils
Virgil Wodicka, Director, Bureau of Foods	came from	Ralston Purina; Libby, McNeill & Libby; Hunt-Wesson
	went to	private consultant to industry
Ogden Johnson, Director, Division of Nutrition	went to	Hershey Co.
Robert Schaffner, Director, Office of Product Technology	came from	Libby, McNeill & Libby
Malcolm Stephens, Assistant Commissioner for Regulations	went to	President, Institute of Shortening and Edible Oils
James Grant, Deputy Commissioner	went to	Special Assistant to the Chairman, CPC International (Skippy peanut butter, Hellmann's mayonnaise, etc.)

| Charles Edwards, Commissioner | came from | Booz, Allen, Hamilton (consulting firm) |
| | went to | Becton, Dickinson & Co. (medical supply co.) |

U.S. Department of Agriculture

Earl Butz, Secretary	came from	Director, Ralston Purina
Clifford Hardin, Secretary	went to	Vice-President and Director, Ralston Purina
Richard Lyng, Assistant Secretary	went to	President, American Meat Institute
Clarence Palmby, Assistant Secretary	went to	Continental Grain Co.
Edward Hekman, Administrator, Food and Nutrition Service	came from	President, Keebler Biscuit Co.; Director, Grocery Manufacturers of America
Robert Long, Assistant Secretary	came from	Bank of America (which has huge land holdings)
Clifford Pulvermacher, Export Marketing Service	went to	Bunge Corp. (grain dealer)
George Shanklin, Assistant Sales Manager of Commodity Exports	went to	Bunge Corp.
Clyde Merriman, Assistant Sales Manager of Commodity Exports	went to	Louis Dreyfus (grain dealer)
Caro Luhrs, M.D., Medical Advisor to the Secretary	went to	Director, Pillsbury Co.
Steven Laine Director of Public Affairs	came from	International Foodservice Manufacturers Association; Cling Peach Advisory Board

References

1. Hearings, Senate Select Committee on Nutrition and Human Needs, December 5, 1972.
2. U.S. Department of Agriculture *Yearbook*, 1959, p. 9.
3. Statistical Bulletin, Metropolitan Life Insurance Co., January, 1960.
4. *Journal of the American Medical Association*, Vol. 221 (1972) p. 579.
5. Hearings, Senate Select Committee on Nutrition and Human Needs, December 19, 1968, p. 153.
6. *Science*, Vol. 185 (1974), p. 932.
7. *Cancer*, Vol. 17 (1964), p. 486.
8. *Advertising Age* (August 26, 1974).
9. Congressional Record, June 30, 1972, p. E6703.
10. Hearings, Senate Commerce Committee, August 4, 1970.
11. *Women's Wear Daily*, January 11, 1974.
12. *Washington Evening Star*, September 22, 1970.
13. M. Jacobson and R. White, "Company Town at FDA," *Progressive*, (April, 1973).
14. *Journal of the American Dietetic Association*, Vol. 38 (1961) p. 27.
15. Hearings, Senate Commerce Committee, July, 1970.
16. *British Journal of Surgery*, Vol. 58 (1971), p. 695.
17. *British Medical Journal*, Vol. 1 (1973), p. 274.

18. *Brit. Med. J.* Vol. 2 (1971), p. 450.

19. *J. Am. Diet. Asso.* Vol. 60 (1972) p. 499.

20. *Lancet*, Vol. 1 (1974), p. 49.

21. *Brit. Med. J.* Vol. 1 (1968), p. 30.

22. *Atherosclerosis*, Vol. 17 (1973), p. 156.

23. *British Journal of Cancer*, Vol. 27 (1973), p. 167.

24. *Gut*, Vol. 14 (1973), p. 69.

25. *National Food Situation*, U.S. Department of Agriculture (February, 1973) p. 20.

26. Historical Statistics of the United States, colonial times to 1957, U.S. Bureau of the Census, 1960, p. 187.

27. Statement at press conference, August 1, 1974, Washington, D.C.

28. Hearings, Senate Select Committee on Nutrition and Human Needs, March 5, 1973.

29. U.S. Department of Agriculture *Yearbook*, 1959, p. 219.

30. National Caries Program, Status Report 1972, National Institute of Dental Research, p. 1.

31. *Annals of Internal Medicine*, Vol. 74 (1971), p. 278.

32. *American Journal of Clinical Nutrition*, Vol. 27 (1974), p. 403.

33. *Lancet*, Vol. 1 (1970), p. 870.

34. Hearings, Senate Select Committee on Nutrition and Human Needs, April 30, 1973.

35. *Ann. Internal Med.* Vol. 62 (1965), p. 1188.

36. *Journal of Comparitive Physiology and Psychology*, Vol. 84 (1973), p. 496.

37. *New England Journal of Medicine*, Vol. 277 (1967), p. 186.

38. *J. Am. Diet. Asso.*, Vol. 52 (1968), p. 202.

39. *Am. J. Clin. Nutr.*, Vol. 25 (1972), p. 1399.

40. *Consumer Reports*, August, 1970.

41. Hearings, House Subcommittee on Livestock and Grains, July 31, 1974.

42. *Statistical Abstract of the United States*, Government Printing Office, Washington, D.C.

43. *Ann. Internal Med.* Vol. 74 (1971), p. 1.

44. American Heart Association Monograph No. 18, 1968.

45. *Lancet*, Vol. 2 (1972), p. 835.

46. J. Stamler, *Lectures on Preventive Cardiology*, (New York, Grune and Stratton, 1967).

47. *Journal of the American Oil Chemists Society*, Vol. 51 (1974) p. 244.

48. Agricultural Economic Report No. 138, Economic Research Service, USDA, Government Printing Office, Washington, D.C. (1968) and subsequent supplements.

49. *Present Knowledge in Nutrition*, 3rd edition (New York, Nutrition Foundation) p. 55.

50. J. C. Drummond, *The Englishman's Food* (London, Jonathan Cape, 1958), p. 467.

51. *Public Health News* (New Jersey), June, 1966, p. 132.

52. L. Pauling, *Vitamin C and the Common Cold* (New York, Bantam, 1971).

53. *Canadian Medical Association Journal*, Vol. 111 (1974), p. 31.

54. Paper presented at the Western Hemisphere Nutrition Congress IV, Bal Harbour, Florida, August 22, 1974.

55. *Present Knowledge in Nutrition*, p. 152.

56. R. J. Williams, *Nutrition Against Disease* (New York, Pitman, 1971), p. 81.

57. *J. Am. Diet. Asso.*, Vol. 59 (1971), p. 212.

58. Paper given at the 1971 annual meeting of the American Association for the Advancement of Science.

59. *Medical Counterpoint*, July, 1971, p. 16.
60. *Pediatrics Research*, Vol. 6, (1972), p. 868.
61. M. Bierenbaum, paper presented at the Western Hemisphere Nutrition Congress IV, Bal Harbour, Florida, August 20, 1974.
62. Complaint sent by Center for Science in the Public Interest to FDA, June, 1974.
63. Data from Food and Drug Administration.
64. Ben F. Feingold, *Why Your Child is Hyperactive* (New York, Random House, 1975).
65. M. Jacobson, *How Sodium Nitrite Can Affect Your Health*, Center for Science in the Public Interest, April, 1973.
66. M. Jacobson, *Eater's Digest* (New York, Doubleday & Co., 1972), p. 89.
67. *ibid*, p. 85.
68. "Fats in Food and Diet," Agriculture Information Bulletin No. 361, USDA, Government Printing Office, Washington, D.C., 1974.
69. *Am. J. Clin. Nutr.*, Vol. 9 (1961), p. 530.
70. *Lancet*, Vol. 1 (1970), p. 870.
71. *Family Health* (November, 1973), p. 24.
72. *New York Times Magazine*, February 25, 1973, p. 14.
73. Prepared statement, Hearings, Panel on Nutrition and Health, Senate Select Committee on Nutrition and Human Needs, June, 1974; pers. comm.
74. *Hypertension*, National Institutes of Health Report No. 1714, Government Printing Office, Washington, D.C., 1969.
75. Second Special Report on Alcohol and Health, National Institute on Alcohol Abuse and Alcoholism, 1974.
76. *Bulletin of the New York Academy of Medicine*, Vol. 47 (1971), p. 569. Speech at La Leche League

International Convention, July 11, 1974, Chicago, Illinois.

77. S. J. Fomon, *Infant Nutrition*, 2nd ed. (Philadelphia, W. B. Saunders, Co., 1974), p. 8.

78. *Washington Post*, December 28, 1972.

79. *New York Times*, July 28, 1973, p. 31.

80. *Proposed Fortification Policy for Cereal-Grain Products*, National Academy of Sciences, Washington, D.C., 1974.

81. *Washington Post*, September 15, 1974.

82. Hearings, Senate Select Committee on Nutrition and Human needs, April, 1973, pp. 559-560.

83. *Acta Odontologica Scandinavica*, Vol. 11 (1954), p. 232.

A Selected Bibliography

America, Inc., Morton Mintz and Jerry Cohen (Dell, 1972). A detailed, carefully documented analysis of corporate power and abuses of that power.

By Bread Alone, Lester Brown (Praeger, 1974). The best, most readable overview of the world food situation.

Chemical Feast, James Turner (Grossman, 1970). An inside glimpse of the Food and Drug Administration.

Diet for a Small Planet, Frances Moore Lappé (Ballantine, 1975). A lucid explanation, from an ecological viewpoint, of why we should be eating more vegetable-based foods.

Eater's Digest, Michael F. Jacobson (Doubleday & Co., 1972). A reliable and critical book on food additives.

Eating May Be Hazardous to Your Health, Jacqueline Verrett and Jean Carper (Simon & Schuster, 1974). An FDA toxicologist gives her view of the FDA.

Eat Your Heart Out, Jim Hightower (Crown Publishers, 1975). The story of agribusiness by someone who has investigated it for the past five years.

Food for People, Not for Profit, ed. Catherine Lerza and Michael F. Jacobson (Ballantine, 1975). An encyclopedic account of problems related to our food supply and what you can do about them.

Recipes for a Small Planet, Ellen Ewald (Ballantine,

1973). An excellent vegetarian cookbook, which uses the principles of mixing proteins, as described in *Diet for a Small Planet.*

Sowing the Wind, Harrison Wellford (Grossman, 1972). A critical, authoritative, in-depth analysis of the Department of Agriculture.

The American Food Scandal, William Robbins (William Morrow & Co., 1974). An excellent description of the abuses of power by agribusiness corporations and food manufacturers.

The Supermarket Handbook, Nikki and David Goldbeck (Harper & Row, 1973). A wealth of information on all kinds of foods and cooking.

The Center for Science in the Public Interest has published a poster and several reports that will be of interest to readers of *Nutrition Scoreboard.* They may be purchased from CSPI-Dept. G, 1779 Church St. NW, Washington, D.C. 20036.

1. *Nutrition Scoreboard poster:* A beautiful 18″ x 24″ color poster with nutritional ratings of over 200 foods and tidbits of nutrition advice. It is perfect for the refrigerator door or classoom wall, and is a great way of getting children to think about nutrition. $1.75 for one poster; $1 each for additional posters.

2. *Food Scorecard:* A booklet intended for children 9-12 years old that makes use of the *Nutrition Scoreboard* food rating system. This delightful 32-page booklet, with illustrations by Kathy Kahn, is a perfect way for teachers to introduce their students to concepts of nutrition. 20-99 copies, 35¢ each; 100-999 copies, 30¢ each.

3. *Scorecard for Better Eating:* A booklet intended for mass distribution in health clinics, doctors' offices,

social welfare offices, and high schools that is appropriate for people of high school age or older. It is illustrated and uses the *Nutrition Scoreboard* rating system. 32 pages. 20-99 copies, 35¢ each; 100-999 copies, 30¢ each.

4. *Creative Food Experiences for Children*, by Mary Goodwin, M.P.H. and Geraldine Pollen: This unique resource book for teachers and parents is a gold mine of activities, games, facts, and recipes designed to make food and nutrition a lively and exciting topic. Focusing on natural foods, it encourages children to use all five senses in exploring foods—not only with nutrition exercises and recipes, but also with activities applicable to science, art, and other subject areas. 8½" x 11", 191 pages, $4.

Index

Disease
    and diet, 6-8, 10, 17, 18-
        20
    and fiber deficiency, 43-45
    and high-fat meat, 57
    see also individual diseases
Drinks
    nutritional contribution of,
        135
    nutritional ratings, 139
Drugs, 70
Drummond, Jack Cecil, 86

*Eating May Be Hazardous to
    Your Health,* 98
Edwards, Charles, 111
Eggs, cholesterol in, 16, 65,
    103-5
Enzymes
    and digestion of milk, 140-
        41
    and magnesium, 90-91
    and zinc deficiency, 95
Ewald, Ellen, 157

Farmer, Jean, 29
Fats
    compared to oils, 67
    content in common foods,
        58-59
    content in meat, 56-57, 60-
        61, 157-58
    formula for rating of, 55
    function of, 67
    how to reduce intake, 56
    nutritional rating of, 66
    relation to disease, 57
    see also Oils; Polyunsatu-
        rated fats; Saturated fats
FDA, *see* Food and Drug Ad-
    ministration
Fertilizers, 106-8
Fiber, dietary
    in diet, 42, 43-45
    and disease, 43-45

sources of, 42-43, 45
    and weight control, 11
Flour, *see* Refined flour;
    Whole wheat
Food additives, 97-102
    see also individual addi-
        tives
Food and Drug Administra-
    tion
    and enriched foods, 161-62
    and food additives, 98-99,
        164
    officials in, 25-26
    and sugared cereals, 175-
        76
Food industry, 26, 28, 51, 60,
    125-56
    advertising campaigns, 11-
        15, 18, 22-23, 29
    and nutrition information,
        10-14, 19-22
Framingham study, 61, 65
Franken-Berry, 176-77
*Free and Inexpensive Educa-
    tion Aids,* 11
Frozen meals rated, 168-70
Fruit, canned, 186
Fruits, fresh, 82
    nutritional ratings, 152-53
    see also individual fruits

Genes, 70

Hambridge, K. Michael, 95
Harris, Robert, 32, 124
Hawkins, David, 155
Health, Education and Wel-
    fare Department, 3, 16,
    85-86
Heart disease, 61, 65
    and cholesterol levels, 16,
        60-66, 103
    and diet, 6, 17, 45, 50, 60-
        67, 95-96
    risk factors, 65-66
Hegsted, D. Mark, 4, 147

209

Nitrosamines, 101, 155-56
Nizel, Abraham, 48-49
Nursing, *see* Breast-feeding
Nutrition
    good, 2, 3, 5, 21, 70, 147
    need for education in, 6,
        10, 11, 13, 14, 16-17, 22
    studies on, 3, 8, 19-22
    see also malnutrition
Nutritional ratings
    explanation of, 127-30
    formula used for, 34-36,
        71, 97, 109, 125-26, 127-
        30, 162
    shortcomings of, 123-26
    use of brand names in,
        129-30
Nuts, 181

Obesity, 110
    and diet, 44, 45, 55, 118
    problem in America, 4, 109
Oils, 67, 102
Orange juice
    nutritional value of, 135,
        139
    substitutes for, 138-39
Oregon, 108
Organic food, 106-8
Oxalic acid, 89
    in vegetables, 89, 145

Panel on Nutrition and
        Health, 8, 10, 72, 112-
        13
Pasta, 164-66
Pauling, Linus, 81
Peas, 146
Pellagra, 79
Pepe, Thomas J., 11
Peterson, Esther, 15
Phytic acid, 8, 162-63
Pickle, 13
Pickle Packers International,
        11, 13
Polatty, Nancy, 128

Polyunsaturated fats, 60-67
    nutritional rating of, 66
Popcorn, 182
Preservatives, 101-3
Proteins
    amino acids in, 37-40
    in dairy products, 140, 142
    effect on certain vitamins,
        72, 79, 92
    formula used for rating, 37
    function of, 37, 153
    Net Protein Utilization
        (NPU), 37-40
    nutritional ratings, 38-40,
        158-59
    RDA, 38
    sources of, 37-40, 140, 142,
        153, 156-57
    in vegetables, 156-57
Pyridoxine, *see* Vitamin B-6

RDA (Recommended Di-
        etary Allowance)
    of carbohydrates, 42n
    and nutrition, 3n
    of protein, 38
    used in formula, 35-36n
Recipes for a Small Planet,
        157
Red No. 2, 99
Refined flour, 44, 90
    disadvantages of, 91, 92,
        94-95
Riboflavin, *see* Vitamin B-2
Rice, 165
    nutritional ratings, 166
    see also Brown rice; White
        rice
Rice and Vegetable Nirvana
        recipe, 148
Romaine, 145
Ross, Warren B., 47
Roughage, *see* Fiber, dietary

Saccharine, 138

A GOURMET'S SELECTION OF COOKBOOKS FROM AVON

THE AMERICAN WOMAN'S COOKBOOK
Ruth Berolzheimer, Ed.   20610   1.95

THE COMPLETE BOOK OF SALADS   Beryl Marton   19265   2.95

THE CONDIMENT COOKBOOK
Heinz   19612   1.25

THE COOK'S COMPANION
Frieda Arkin   12799   2.95

THE FRUIT COOKBOOK
Suzanne Topper   14803   2.95

THE GOOD HOUSEKEEPING INTERNATIONAL COOKBOOK   10041   1.25

THE NATURAL BABY FOOD COOKBOOK   Margaret Elizabeth
Kenda and Phyllis S. Williams   21170   1.25

THE NEW YORK TIMES NATURAL FOODS COOKBOOK
Jean Hewitt   12468   1.95

THE NATURALLY GOOD WHEAT GERM COOKBOOK
Kretschmer   19794   1.25

THE TOO-GOOD-TO-BE-LEFTOVERS COOKBOOK
Hellmann's/Best Foods   18325   1.25

THE WEST AFRICAN COOK BOOK   Ellen Gibson Wilson   13201   3.95

ZEN MACRIOBIOTIC COOKING
Michel Abehsera   09563   1.25

Available wherever paperbacks are sold, or directly from the publisher. Includes 25¢ per copy for mailing; allow three weeks for delivery. Avon Books, Mail Order Dept., 250 West 55th Street, New York, N.Y. 10019.

GC 10-75